Also by Bobbi Giudicelli
(aka Joanne K Giudicelli)

Hire Power: A Radical New Strategy for Defining
and Executing Successful Hiring

Freedom
FROM A TOXIC
RELATIONSHIP WITH
Food

A JOURNEY THAT WILL GIVE YOU YOUR LIFE BACK

COPYRIGHT

To my three sons,
Michael, Christopher and Bryan,
who are a big part of everything I do, always!

To Roger who learned how to handle my stress
as I wrote this book.

I love you for not running away.

"If you want to find a better path, you have to be willing to explore a different path."

- James Clear,
author of Atomic Habits

"Let food be thy medicine and medicine be thy food."

- Hippocrates

CONTENTS

ACKNOWLEDGEMENTS

My life wouldn't be nearly as joyful if it weren't for Roger, Michael, Christopher and Bryan, the four most special men with whom I have the privilege of sharing so much. You all have played such a big part in who I am today, and you've been the joy in my life for the last three-plus decades.

Michael, a special thank you for your trust in me to be my business partner and co-founder of Read The Ingredients. You really are the best business partner I've ever had.

To my dear aunt, Ellin Blumenthal. While we didn't know each other until my early 20s, I was fortunate enough to have you as my 'chosen mother' for the past 45 years. You've consistently and unconditionally given me more love, support and acknowledgment than anybody. You certainly provided me with the role model I needed to become the mom I am.

Thank you, Patricia Hurley, for being such a big part of this journey and so many other aspects of my life for the past 13 years. You really are my sister from another mother, and we both drew the short straw in the mother department.

Donna Liebert, while the angels were looking out for me, they reconnected us after 45 years. I know we'll be there for each other for the next 45.

This book has been brewing in me for the past six years. I never thought I'd get a chance to write it, thereby keeping the promise I made to myself many years ago. Mitali Deypurkaystha, I believe it was fate that had our paths cross. If it weren't for that, this book wouldn't be. You're a very special woman, and you do not give yourself the credit you deserve for how special you are. I look forward to keeping in touch beyond publication.

To those special friends (and family) who were willing to read the early versions of this book, I'm forever grateful. You helped make it a better read. Many thanks to Melissa Lyster, Carmen Rogers, Sasha Tannenbaum, Judi Mosley, Katie Carter, Sheryl Lynde, Hana Bowers, Patricia Hurley and Donna Liebert.

PREFACE

Like so many others, I'd spent many years in pursuit of thinness. I'd no idea of the external forces at play that had me fail in my efforts to lose weight and keep it off. I had no idea about the concept expressed in the famous Hippocrates quote, "Let food be thy medicine and medicine be thy food."

When I started my journey to learn about and adopt a healthy nutritional diet ten years ago and learned what I now know, I discovered that it's all about my individual relationship with food and the foods I choose to eat. I want to share with you a little about my life and my recent ten-year journey to a better, healthier lifestyle. Mostly, I want to share with you how you, too, can gain freedom from a toxic relationship with food and get your life back.

If you're reading this book, then I'm sure I've walked at least one mile in your shoes. I've spent 40 years pursuing a healthy relationship with food. Wait a minute. That's not exactly an honest statement. The reality is that I've spent most of those years desperate to lose weight, so I'd look good. I believed that in itself would make my life better. It's a more honest statement to say that I've spent the best part of 40 years using food for things other than health. And, I tried very hard to stay thin while doing it. Needless to say, I wasn't successful until it became about my health and *not* about my weight.

I'm not a doctor, I'm not a professional nutritionist, and I'm absolutely not a celebrity. I am an ordinary, albeit very driven woman who has realized many of her dreams and goals throughout her life while feeling good about my body and appearance had constantly eluded me.

I want to share my journey, and I believe, in doing so I can help lots of people like me. Every step of my journey was taken after I dug in and did the research for myself. The irony is that by the time I seriously started this journey to a healthy relationship with food, I felt so physically tired that the concern about weight loss was not a motivating factor at all. I just wanted to find some energy and get my life back.

In the introduction, I share a summary of my life story, so you'll understand that your struggles are not unique. I never believed I'd be in the position to write this book. Whether you see your challenge as wanting to lose and maintain a healthy weight once and for all, or you realize that you don't have a healthy relationship with food, I've written this book to take this journey with you.

While I was learning about food and how to have a better relationship with it, I was careful to understand the research sources I was reviewing. It was important to recognize unbiased versus biased sources of information. The food industry is huge. Their job is to sell you food. The research they provide is often not reliable. For example, Coca-Cola has been known to research the effects of sugar. They have documented research[1] that indicates sugar isn't so bad for you. The egg industry likewise has sponsored studies[2] that have concluded that the fat in eggs does not impact your cholesterol. In both cases, unbiased studies[3] show the opposite. Remember the tobacco industry studies[4] in the second half of the 1900s?

The diet industry is huge too. Their job is to sell you books, consulting services and diet-specific foods, so the 'evidence' they provide that their diets work are often unreliable. I'm curious about what motivated you to read this book. I hope you know going forward that this is *not* a diet book. It's a book about your health and your overall quality of life.

If you're reading this book with your motivation being your struggle to lose weight, that's perfect. You're right where you need to be. If you're reading this book with the motivation to feel strong, more energized, and healthier, that's perfect. You're right where you need to be.

If you're reading this book with the motivation to transition to a Whole-Food Plant-Based (WFPB) way of eating and you're looking for some support and suggestions, please keep reading. You're right where you need to be.

Perhaps you've been diagnosed with cancer, heart disease, diabetes, auto-immune diseases or other diseases and you're lucky enough to have received advice that a change in food choices can help to reverse your disease or prevent it from getting worse. In that case, you're right where you need to be. And I'm sorry that it took a BBE (Big Bad Event) for you to realize the opportunity.

I wrote this book to help you on your journey. Regardless of what motivated you to pick up this book, you can successfully accomplish your goals by creating a healthy, exciting relationship with food. The journey, my journey, presented here, will get you there.

I suggest you only proceed with turning the page if you're not just ready but completely committed to changing your relationship with food. If you want to stop thinking about your weight when you get dressed in the morning, planning your weekend activities or vacation, figuring out what to prepare for dinner, or going to the grocery store, then please continue.

Only read this book, if you want to get your life back, for however long you may live.

INTRODUCTION

"And once the storm is over, you won't remember how you made it through, how you managed to survive. You won't even be sure whether the storm is really over. But one thing is certain. When you come out of the storm, you won't be the same person who walked in. That's what this storm's all about."

— Haruki Murakami

Many people spend their lives bombarded with messages about how to be thin, how to be healthy, and how to look good. Try this diet, cut out drinking, eat more slowly, use a smaller plate, and so on. Many of these suggestions do come with rules, and usually the suggestion is just to follow these rules until you reach some particular goal. Then good for you, go celebrate! You go shopping for smaller clothes or go out to dinner with a friend, just to find that the new clothes don't fit so well a couple of weeks later.

If you're one of the very slim (no pun intended) number of dieters who have found success following the rules, you can stop reading now. If you're able to maintain your weight and health goals, you're pleased with your relationship with food, and you feel the level of energy you expect, you can close this book.

However, if you're like the rest of us, you're tired of the see-saw dieting, you're tired of being tired, and you're tired of worrying about what you eat for too many hours of the day, then I'm thrilled that you found this book. Keep reading. I'm honored to share my journey with you, and I hope after you've read this book, you'll share your journey with me.

This is *not* another diet book, I promise you. It's a how-to book to create your personal journey that frees you from a toxic relationship with food and guides you toward a healthy relationship with food with more inherent rewards than you can imagine.

ABOUT ME

I'm somewhat of an introvert, and I never languish in self-indulgence, so writing about myself makes me somewhat uncomfortable. However, I felt that sharing my story is important to let you know that I've likely been there, whatever your starting point is.

I was brought into this world by a biological mother who was diagnosed schizophrenic. By the time I was born, her illness was in full bloom. She was in no position to nurture or parent my sister or me. I was bottle-fed and most likely lacked any real maternal bond. I bring this up because, for many years, I was confident that my food issues had something to do with the lack of nurturing and the fact that I was bottle-fed. Now, I'm not so sure, and it's no longer of any interest to me to figure out.

My parents divorced when I was five years old. My father got custody of us. For a couple of years, any mother figure was absent from our lives. My father married my stepmother, Sandy, when I was seven years old. When we were introduced to her, I was thankful to have a mother and finally have our family look like other families. In retrospect,

I realize Sandy came to the family with her eating disorders, two children (my step-siblings), and a raging temper that she let loose on me frequently within the first 12 months they were married. She remained physically abusive toward me for the next nine years.

Sandy met my father when she was 27. She came to our home addicted to diet pills to keep herself thin. She was attractive, vain, and very unhealthy. Our typical family dinners would consist of a meat and potatoes meal that my father insisted on while she'd serve herself half a grapefruit. Clearly, I had a role model that taught me that being thin was important. When I turned 17 and thought I was over-weight, which I wasn't, I got my hands on diet pills and learned to count calories obsessively.

My father had a personality disorder as well. He was a classic narcissist. As such, my father turned a blind eye to anything that didn't suit him, make him look good, or was out of his control. He was a stickler for the rules he set, and this was especially true at the dinner table. We had to eat what was served to us, all of it, and we were required to demonstrate impeccable table manners. Dinner time, and food in general, were unpleasant.

My sister Ronnie, who was 17 months older, was very rebellious. We were anything but close, and our relationship was always contentious. In fact, by the time we were in our late teens, we couldn't be in the same room for more than 15 minutes without arguing. We finally became close for the last year and a half of her life as she slowly died of ovarian cancer. I became one of her primary caregivers and spent that time frequently crossing the country from my home in California to hers in Florida.

While my sister's survival mechanism included rebellious behavior, physically and emotionally escaping, I took on the 'good girl' and overachiever role. I later found out these are often traits of someone who develops eating disorders. I was a straight-A student in school, and I was sure to do everything and anything I thought would get me noticed or loved, but to no avail. I finally left home in 11th grade.

I developed a concern for my weight in my senior year of high school. Ronnie and I were built differently. She was just under 5ft 2in (1.57m) and weighed about 112lb (51kg). In contrast, I was 5ft 8in (1.72m) and weighed appropriately 140lb (64kg). While I wanted to be inconspicuous because of my horrible shyness and low self-esteem, I felt everyone saw me as a big blob.

Shortly after moving out of my parent's home, a doctor prescribed me diet pills, and I got hooked instantly. The pills created an incredible feeling of conquering the world. My appetite for food disappeared. After three months, the doctor told me he wouldn't renew the prescription. I don't remember how much weight I had lost, but I know I'd lost a fair amount. Once the pills were out of my system, I remember sleeping for the next ten days. I was voraciously hungry and quickly put the lost weight back on. Being self-conscious about my weight and my body continued to plague me.

At 18, I went off to college and discovered starvation. My best friend at school and I were both conscious of not gaining the 'freshman 15' (an American expression to explain the expectation that girls will gain 15lb after going off to college). There were times we'd go to the dorm dining hall for dinner and eat only carrots dipped in salad dressing. We'd eat enough carrots to turn our hands orange. We were confident that we'd found the secret to weight maintenance and shared the idea with many girls in our dorm.

However, the most brilliant move came when I was on vacation with my then-boyfriend, later my first of three husbands. I decided if I had the willpower to pass on breakfast and lunch, I could reward myself with eating whatever I wanted for dinner, including dessert. That worked well enough until I started to think that I was still overweight. How about if I eat less for dinner and skip dessert? How about if I eat iceberg lettuce with lemon juice as my whole dinner? That will fill me up, and I'll finally get to be thin. That's how I became a full-fledged anorexic. I told myself I just needed to walk down the aisle three years later, looking thin. Mission accomplished.

After several solid years of starving myself and getting my weight to a low of 104lb (47kg), something in me snapped. The anorexia transitioned to bulimia. Once an anorexic starts eating, it's hard to stop. I remember thinking that binging and purging was a brilliant discovery. I could eat what I wanted and get it out of my system before the calories could land fat everywhere on my body. If I felt the purging wasn't working well enough, I'd take double or triple doses of laxatives.

When I was 34 years old and my third son was born, I decided I couldn't do this anymore. After 14 years of bulimic behavior, I was going to find out how to control myself around food and set an example for my children. It was much easier said than done for all the reasons I'll discuss in this book.

I'd spent 16 years living dangerously with eating disorders, and for the entire time, I went out of my way to hide this from everyone. Back then, nobody talked about eating disorders. It was a shameful, lonely disease. I was defeated, depressed, and felt completely out of control around food. I committed to discontinuing the binging and purging, but I only gave up the purging in reality. Binging, starving, counting calories and being extremely unhappy with how I looked and felt became my reality for another 20 years. I tried Overeaters Anonymous, individual therapy, and several group therapy sessions. It always came down to my weight and feeling fat and ugly. How could I be so accomplished in other areas of my life and yet feel unable to control my weight?

I was determined to maintain a set weight, even though 160-168lb (73-76kg) was still heavier than I liked my weight to be. There have been many times I've looked for the answer in prescribed diets, even when they haven't worked before. Why would I think they'd suddenly work now? The definition of insanity is doing the same thing again and expecting different results. Fortunately, I liked to exercise. I maintained a level of activity that meant I didn't gain weight. But exercise alone couldn't help me lose weight.

Nothing seemed to do the trick. There were many times over the early years that I explored the psychological reasons why I couldn't lose weight. I reflected on growing up in such a dysfunctional home. In retrospect, there was some solace in feeling like I could pass the responsibility and blame onto someone else. But blaming others doesn't solve the problem. Addressing the problem head-on solves the problem.

MY JOURNEY BEGINS

Finally, about ten years ago, well into my 50s, my journey to a healthy lifestyle and healthy eating began.

Three events motivated me. The first was when Ronnie was diagnosed with ovarian cancer at age 50. She was treated and in remission for a year and a half. When her cancer returned, I volunteered to be her primary caregiver. I spent three weeks of every month in Florida. Ronnie was dying a slow, painful death, and it was tough to watch. I'm so embarrassed to say this but seeing my sister in the emaciated state of a dying woman made me feel even more conscious of my weight. How embarrassing is that to say out loud? I now know there is a connection between cancer and diet, and when I discovered that, a lightbulb went on.

The second of three events was related to my father. I saw and talked to him more during the last years of Ronnie's life. It was becoming apparent that this man who had skied, ridden bikes, played tennis, and was quite active until age 80 was quickly losing his ability to do any of that physically or mentally. He was diagnosed and medicated for heart disease that he'd suffered from for more years than I knew. He also clearly had very progressive dementia. Several episodes put him into the hospital, and for the next two years, I was again flying coast to coast to help him. When he died at 91 years old, I thought if I was going to live to my 90s, which I likely will, I didn't want to have my quality of life deteriorate as my dad's had for the last ten years of his life.

The third event, and the one that left me no choice, was my own chronic fatigue. I'd started noticing a significant decline in my energy at the age of 40. When I brought this up to my doctor, she'd always explain it away by saying this is normal when you're getting older. I'd been in my 40s then. By my 50s, the fatigue was so bad there were days I could barely walk the length of my property without resting.

For the first time in my life, I was more concerned about my health than my weight. These things led me to the journey I describe in this book, which literally gave me my life back.

I got into taking action with my own research. I've never trusted doctors much as I've had some negative and scary experiences with mistreatment and misdiagnoses of serious situations. While I was learning what I needed to do to feel better, I kept coming back to the fact that longevity runs in my family. I want to have a good quality of life and be independent and active as long as I live. I was determined to understand not just how to be healthy at my current age, but at any age.

Full disclosure. Today, I eat 95% whole foods and 100% plant-based foods. I feel great, and my weight is back down to the 140lb (64kg) that I weighed in high school (my correct weight). I love eating, and I love food more today than I ever have in my entire life. I miss none of the foods I used to eat. I love the exploration of new foods. I love going to the grocery store, cooking and preparing meals. These are two things that not only didn't interest me but actually scared me in the past. Ironically, I raised my three boys with my husband, Roger, doing all of the cooking and grocery shopping. I often think about what could have been if I'd started this journey earlier. Then I realized each of our paths in life happens exactly when and how they should with opportunities presented and lessons learned.

Are you ready to take this journey of self-love and compassion and free yourself from a toxic relationship with food, once and for all? I promise I'll hold your hand along the way, and then some.

THE IRONY OF MY LIFE JOURNEY

There is an irony to my life's journey that I'd like to share. I'm a serial entrepreneur. I've founded and built several different companies.

Ironically, five years before I started this journey, I founded a wholesale and retail frozen yogurt business as one of the first self-serve frozen yogurt retail shops. It absolutely tested how far I'd come from the days of binging and purging. I spent many years avoiding working in the food industry because I didn't trust myself around food.

The second irony was that I'd always questioned how I could be someone who seems to accomplish whatever I set my mind to, except for my previously toxic relationship with food and my ability to attain and maintain my perfect weight. One of the goals that drove me from a young age was to be a mom, and unlike how I was raised, have a great relationship with my kids. I have three sons who I adore, and they're all married with families of their own. We're all quite close, while only one son's family lives nearby. This son is my business partner today. We built the yogurt business together, and we're co-founders of our current company, Read The Ingredients, also a food business. We've created some of the healthiest packaged foods on the market. Read The Ingredients was born from our respective journeys and the need to take better care of ourselves through discovering how to eat (more about this later).

I said many years ago that if I could just lose the weight, life would be great, and I'd have it all. I had no idea that it wasn't about the weight. The rest of the statement, it turns out, is true. Yes, I now have my health, my loving family, a business we're passionate about, my animals and a great relationship with food. I do feel like I have it all.

WHY I'M WRITING THIS BOOK

A big part of eating disorders is the distorted reality about my body (body dysmorphia) and food. Shame, loneliness and isolation. I experienced it all in the '70s and '80s when I first discovered how to starve myself. I was sure that my chances of being 'cured' were pretty slim. I thought the best I could hope for was that I'd be strong enough to control my weight one day.

I'd promised myself back then that if I ever did develop a healthy relationship with food, I'd figure out a way to pay it forward. This book, and the company I co-founded with my son, Michael, are my way of paying it forward. I'm committed to helping others who find themselves in the same situation.

FOR WHOM AM I WRITING THIS BOOK

This book is for anybody who has struggled in their relationship with food. That may be overeaters and bingers. It may be people who can't figure out why they can't lose those extra pounds. It's for people who use and maybe abuse substances or unhealthy foods and aren't living a healthy life. It's also for people who want to roll the dice in their favor against genetically predisposed diseases.

The other audience that I'd hope to reach with this book is those struggling with heart disease, cancer, diabetes, autoimmune diseases, etc. I feel that I'm honoring my sister's legacy by reflecting on my time as her caregiver because that was a significant motivating factor in the launch of my journey. I'm desperate to share what I didn't know when my sister was suffering and what too many doctors don't seem to know. The Standard American Diet (SAD) is made up of unhealthy, highly processed food, and it's been shown to impact many diseases. In contrast, healthy food has been shown to reverse these diseases. I know I will have more credibility with people who have struggled with their weight than I will with those afflicted with diseases while their doctors are treating them with drugs. Therefore, if you have loved ones who are ill, I encourage you to share this message with them. As defined in this book, the combination of healthy eating and doctor-recommended treatments should be considered in their battle against these conditions.

WHAT THIS BOOK COVERS

The journey for me started with taking action and educating myself simultaneously. I'll explore both with you.

First, I'll lay the groundwork for you to understand what your relationship with food looks like and how you got there. Let's look at how you went from a baby that eats when you're hungry and stops when satisfied to a teenager and adult whose relationship with food has morphed into something much more complex (and possibly toxic).

Then let's examine the psychology of eating, explore why the 'diets' you've tried don't work and the fact that they prioritize your weight over your health. You'll discover the craziness of diets that many have tried repeatedly and failed more times than most can remember.

Next, I'll share what I've learned about food and nutrition that will help you understand why this journey will take you exactly where you want to be. I'll highlight information that I deeply researched while a novice in nutritional awareness. From this research, I gained an understanding of why most people are fighting a losing battle with their weight their entire lives. This must be understood to make good choices moving forward.

And finally, I'll share what the journey from a toxic relationship to a healthy relationship with food looks like and my personal journey that has given me my life back!

Please note. Occasionally I quote from studies that I've researched to support what I'm saying. These are annotated with numbered references detailed in the Endnotes section at the back of the book.

RESOURCES

This journey can sometimes feel challenging and overwhelming. I wrote this book to help you get your life back. While there are a lot of books that explain the science behind the information I share, I wanted this book to be emotional support for those ready to proceed on their own journey.

I realize that some don't need to do a bunch of research, but others are more analytical and want to dig into the weeds. If the latter sounds like you, there is a Resources section at the back of the book. It includes sources of information from experts who helped me understand the science and much of what helped me figure out this journey. I also suggest exercises at the end of each chapter. These are designed to help you pinpoint the toxic elements of your relationship with food and how you will overcome them.

LET'S GO!

If you're committed to developing a healthy relationship with food and all that it offers, if you really want to stop complaining about your weight, letting it drive your mood every day, or stop wondering why you're so tired and achy all the time, you've come to the right place. I hope that you feel supported all the way through. If you're ready with all the enthusiasm and courage, it takes to make life-altering changes, let's breathe, let's commit, and let's go on the journey that will give you your life back!

"In any given moment, we have two options: to step forward into growth or step back into safety."

—Abraham Maslow

CHAPTER I

HOW WE GOT HERE

"A person's relationship with food is one of their most important relationships."

—Ned Vizzini

INTRODUCTION

This chapter will look at what is meant when talking about a 'relationship with food.' Let's examine why so many people are obsessed with their weight and explore the idea that no one really chooses the food they eat. Yes, really. It may be that the big food companies are making those choices *for* us.

To accomplish anything in life, you must want it badly enough, and you should have your actions be consistent with reaching the goal. That's certainly true of your goal to build a healthy relationship with food. I intended this book to not only help you succeed in that goal but also be thought-provoking. I hope that this journey expands beyond the relationship with food and encourages you to look at other areas of your life where you may want to make changes.

RELATIONSHIPS

The definition of relationship is:

- the way in which two or more concepts, objects, or people are connected, or the state of being connected
(Oxford English Dictionary)

Most relationships are fresh and exciting initially, with all kinds of possibilities. Once the relationship is established, and past the newness, there are always ups and downs. It seems no relationship ever appears perfect. You work on the parts of the relationship that don't seem to be going so well, or you 'settle' for a mediocre relationship (or worse), or you may decide to terminate the relationship. This is true whether talking about relationships with people or objects.

RELATIONSHIPS WITH PEOPLE

Let's, for example, consider relationships with friends and family. When you meet people, you choose whether to pursue a relationship with that person or not. That relationship could be a potential friend, a family member, a primary partner, or a co-worker. In the beginning, you explore what you have in common. You consider if it'll be a relationship that offers companionship to do shared activities or if it'll be a deeper, emotionally supportive relationship. Finally, you set certain expectations that the relationship will be mutually beneficial and balanced. These factors will affect how you feel about your relationship with another person. This is a concept that you've probably given considerable thought to at different times in your life. Too often, you do not do an actual assessment, and then you find you're in an unsatisfying, unhealthy relationship. At that point, you make a choice.

Do you settle for what you have, work on making it better, or terminate the relationship?

RELATIONSHIP WITH OUR POSSESIONS

Now let's look at people's relationship with things, for example, cars. You know the high most people feel when they get a new car. Wow! You're over the moon excited. You treat it like it's your newborn baby, especially when you first drive it off the lot. You park in the most isolated parking spot in a garage to prevent anyone from breathing on it, let alone possibly scratching it. Then fast-forward a couple of weeks, and this baby gets that first scratch. It gets dirty, and the inside is cluttered with what you need to take with you every day. And, oh no, it has some annoying problems and needs to go back into the shop. Are you not feeling so good about your car anymore? Are you considering getting rid of it and taking an Uber wherever you go?

Whoa, what happened to the high of the new car smell? You have a choice to make. You can choose to wash it on the outside, clean out the inside, and get it to the shop for repairs or a tune-up. It's now almost as good as new, apart from that scratch. How badly does that bother you? Does it drive you crazy, or do you see it as part of the settling-in process? Is your car more comfortable to drive to places because you have less anxiety about the next scratch? After all, you're just starting to make it yours, with the radio stations set as you want them, the seat adjusted perfectly for those long drives, and you know where all the buttons are and how to work the in-dash computer.

Would you want to throw that away, or does it make sense to work on the relationship, so you still feel good about the car you have? Do you tell yourself it'd take too much time to get it back to the 'like new' condition? Or, are you willing to say it's just a car and drive around with it dirty most of the time? That's 'settling' and the path of least resistance. There are advantages to an established relationship, even though it doesn't feel as fresh and perfect as it seemed in the beginning.

It's the same with our homes. Think about where you live. Do you look forward to coming home? Do you feel comfortable in your home? Is it warm and cozy, or cold and sterile? Is it sparsely decorated or rather cluttered? Are you friends with others in the neighborhood? You have a relationship with the place you call home, and that relationship is tied to the feelings you have when you're spending time there. Like your car, if your home isn't as cozy as you'd like, or you don't feel the sense of community you'd strive for, you can choose to make changes. Or you can tell yourself it's not that important and settle for the home where you live. Or you can decide to move and live somewhere else.

I suggest you try to identify precisely how you feel when you get in your car or walk into your home. Imagine it right now. That's what you call a relationship, and yes, it's your choice if you'll make it better, settle for where it is now, or terminate the relationship and move on.

YOUR RELATIONSHIP WITH FOOD

While you probably haven't thought about it in these terms, you also have a relationship with food. Most people think about food as something you eat and need to survive. While this is indeed true, it's not that simple. In caveman days, it was simple. They ate what they could get their hands on. It was all strictly to survive.

Most people aren't aware of their unique relationship with food. Think about how you feel when you're around food at the grocery store or when you open your refrigerator or pantry. Think about your reaction to sitting down at the table with friends or family to eat a meal prepared for you. Do you have the same feelings regardless of what specific food is in front of you? Do you always get excited at the prospect of eating, or does it depend on how hungry you are? Maybe it depends on what you ate earlier that day or how tight your clothes feel? Factors that determine your emotional reaction to food in different scenarios are analogous to the scratches on your car or the color the walls are painted in your house. The only difference is that you can choose to settle for, fix, or terminate your relationship with your car or home. But with food, your choices are limited to settling or fixing.

I suggest fixing the relationship is the way to go. Your relationship with food isn't temporary. It'll be a part of who you are for the rest of your life. It will determine so many things about how you live and feel. Food is in your life to stay. Now that you're thinking about it, haven't you been settling for the relationship that you've created? Doesn't it make sense to fix an unhealthy or toxic relationship with food and replace it with a good, healthy one? I believe the answer is a resounding yes! This is the real 'why' for writing this book.

THE RELATIONSHIP IS CREATED WHEN BORN

Your relationship with food starts with how you were fed as a baby. Within the first few weeks, you're creating your relationship with food. You're born with basic survival instincts, including hunger. Mother Nature equipped your mother with breast milk, the perfect food to feed you. It

> Our ability to make food choices that will offer us control of our future weight, health and appetite has been impacted by what our mothers and care-takers fed us as children.

boosted your immune system and gave you the nutrients you needed to grow in that first four to six months of life. In a perfect world, every baby would be fed from their mothers' breasts. However, we don't live in a perfect world.

Once you're weaned off breast milk and ready to eat solid foods, all bets are off. This is where the relationship with food can go wrong for most people.

Too often, it has become a part of parenting to use food as a reward. "If you eat everything on your plate, you can have ice cream for dessert." Wait. So if you overeat what you're served for dinner, you're rewarded with *more* overeating. Not only that, the reward is unhealthy food. It defies all logic. Additionally, food is too often used as punishment. As a child, who hasn't heard, "Go to your room without dinner?" This approach to raising our children defies all logic.

Were you fed in a nurturing way? Is the environment around the dinner table in your house a positive one? Are you engaging with family members or friends over food? Are you focused on the food, or are you focused on the company? Are you watching TV or working on tomorrow's projects if you're eating alone? How have you chosen to prepare your food? How have you decided what you're eating? All these things contribute to or result from your relationship with food.

FOODS FROM OUR CHILDHOOD

As this relationship starts with your parents or caregivers, many food choices are influenced by foods with sentimental attachment. Often this comes from your family's ethnic or cultural roots. If you grow up in a positive, loving home, then you'll naturally find comfort in foods you were fed as a child, regardless of whether they're good for you or not. If your mother served you cake or ice cream to cheer you up, it might be hard not to yearn for those foods when you're sad. You'll explore this further in Chapter II when discussing why you eat.

CAN YOU REALLY CHANGE YOUR RELATIONSHIP WITH FOOD?

Your relationship with food lives on a spectrum. Eating disorders sit on the far left of the spectrum (strong negative), all the way to the far right, where you have the possibility of the relationship with food that I have today. That is one of joy, pleasure, health and vitality.

EATING DISORDERS

Eating disorders are genuine mental illnesses and disorders that are very dangerous. Eating disorders go far beyond a bad relationship with food. Other psychiatric disorders usually go hand-in-hand with eating disorders such as OCD, anxiety disorder, clinical depression, substance addiction and abuse, etc. While I spent many years struggling with and suffering from anorexia and bulimia, it's beyond the scope of this book to deal with true eating disorders.

If those with eating disorders are fortunate enough to recover from that extreme behavior, they'll have to develop a healthy relationship with food. Once recovery begins, the individual realizes they have an overwhelming fear of food. They'll have to learn how to eat without their brain kicking in with all the signals that they're fighting. In this very dark relationship with food, you can't minimize the struggle to convince the brain that food is a good thing.

At 34 years old, after 16 years of bulimic behavior, I was pregnant with my third son. My pregnancies (with each of my children) had been a motivator to eat without worrying about my weight because, for me, it was more important that I not put my unborn child at risk. Knowing that I'd try to focus on eating well for the next nine months, I made the conscious decision that I'd never purge again.

DISORDERED EATING

Unlike eating disorders, disordered eating isn't necessarily considered a mental illness. It's suggested that overeating (without true binging or purging), constant dieting, under-eating to achieve a specific goal (possibly related to weight or athletic performance), and regularly eating in the absence of hunger are all considered disordered eating. At 34, my behavior around food moved from an eating disorder to disordered eating.

Many people struggle with disordered eating. This may be what made you pick up this book. I'd never thought of it in these terms. It made more sense to me that I was struggling to improve my relationship with food, and for many years it was tied to my quest to be 'thin.'

At 34, I was suddenly on a mission to figure out how to eat the most food with the least number of calories. My goal at that time was to quit putting my fingers down my throat. I was *terrified* of the prospect of getting fat.

The next couple of years were still quite challenging. I no longer allowed myself to live by the rules I'd spent many years and much energy establishing, and I had to make new ones. My old rules were don't eat unless absolutely necessary, and if you do eat, only eat low-calorie foods. If I ended up eating bad foods or too much food (or both, which was usually the case), I would purge ASAP.

Some of the new rules I created were not eating three days a week, eating healthy two days a week, and eating whatever I wanted at the weekend. I can honestly say now that 'whatever I want' translated to the unhealthiest foods I'd been 'using' for many years. Sadly, I didn't understand the definition of 'want.' I had no idea what foods I 'wanted,' or, more accurately, what my body wanted. It was a tall, dangerous order for me.

The reality was that I wasn't really making food choices. The food was choosing and controlling me. My relationship with food was more hate than love. I was proud of myself for terminating my purging behavior, but I didn't enjoy food at all. If I ate healthy, low-calorie foods, I felt pride in my willpower and discipline, but I didn't enjoy eating. I felt guilt and shame if I treated myself to something crazy like chocolate. It didn't help that I justified, not just a piece of chocolate, but at times, an extra-large chocolate bar. Sometimes that meant several extra-large chocolate bars. I was afraid to go into the grocery store. I hated being in the kitchen cooking. I got anxious just opening my refrigerator. What kind of relationship is that? I had less disdain for my first marriages, and I chose to leave them behind. My mantra seemed to be, "If I had willpower and discipline, I'd be thin." I never stopped beating myself up or making excuses for seemingly lacking both.

> ### 💣 Warning:
>
> For the sake of your self-confidence and sanity, limit your exposure to social media.
>
> Recently, studies have been conducted inside Facebook about the impact of their sites on their users. The study specifically called out Instagram's negative impact on young women's body image, eating disorders and depression.
>
> Social media has compounded the problems that existed for many years behind closed doors.

BODY IMAGE

Your relationship with food is also impacted by the myth of the 'perfect body.' You're convinced it's not the one you see in the mirror. This perfect body is presented in every company's attempt to market clothes, food, activities, cars, and everything else. You've relied on what you see around you to determine what the perfect body looks like from a young age. This is society telling you what you should look like and that you could have more fun skiing or feel better driving that car if you looked like that. Ugh!

To make it worse, you don't get an honest answer about how to get there. In fact, nothing about what you're told you should look like is honest. You watch beauty pageants and bodybuilding contests. You go into the grocery store and look at magazine covers with models who are someone's definition of beautiful. We've seen the look and the body so many times that we've, consciously or subconsciously, adopted this as our definition of beautiful.

Ironically, because of technological capabilities, even models and celebrities on magazine covers don't look like this in real life. Would you open a fashion magazine if a heavyset woman was on the cover? Out of curiosity, possibly, but not for information on how to look like her.

I know lately that more and more brands are trying to give equal time to the heavyset woman. I appreciate that the intention is to reduce the incidences of horrible body shaming, sending a message that relieves women from the pressure and unhealthy experience of yoyo dieting. However, I also believe it sends another message that's not so positive. It tells you that you're off the hook when it comes to taking responsibility for your health. It's *not* the weight or appearance that's the problem here. You're at a much higher risk of health complications and disease if you're overweight.

The same magazines sporting covers with perfect body specimens advertise whatever food brand pays them indiscriminately. They use terms that have lost all meaning but convince us that their products are natural, organic, and other commonly used terms that imply their products are healthy. These terms are often misleading, and the products are often unhealthy. The truth is that these labels can appear on heavily processed foods.

Finally, some people try to convince themselves that the answer lies in loving yourself and loving your body. This oversimplifies the problem, especially when your body isn't serving you. Unless you're healthy and have the energy to live your life, it's hard to feel good about your body. As you'll explore in the coming chapters, that isn't possible without a healthy relationship with food.

BIG FOOD COMPANIES EQUALS BIG BUCKS MARKETING

Food packaging and advertising are designed to make you believe positive things about the food being sold. Therefore, it's often quite misleading. The big food companies don't want you to know that living in a capitalist society means big bucks drive big companies to market their products to you. They do this by sending subliminal messages in the ads they run. They have messages and graphics on the packaging, leading you to believe that you're eating something healthy, or that will give you energy, or will help you lose weight, or whatever message they want us to receive.

WHAT'S NEXT

Now that you understand what a relationship with food is and the basic reasons why these relationships are not ideal, it's time to examine all the elements of why and how you choose what you eat.

In Chapter II, you'll look at the emotional side of eating. Let's look at the idea that you eat for reasons other than hunger, and you choose foods for reasons besides health. When you become more aware of why you're eating and what you eat, it'll become clear why you may not have a handle on your weight and health and why you may have a toxic relationship with food. Let's lay the groundwork that allows you to understand that no one fails at diets. It's more likely that diets fail you.

> *"The way you eat is inseparable from your core beliefs about being alive. Your relationship with food is an exact mirror of your feelings about love, fear, anger, meaning and transformation."*
>
> —Geneen Roth

CHAPTER I EXERCISE:

Write the answers to the following questions and post them where they'll be visible to you. It may be helpful to move it to a different spot every couple of days, so you're engaged with your commitment to yourself.

1. What are the top three motivators for you to take this journey to a better relationship with food?

2. What activities have you been avoiding based on your relationship with food?

3. What would you look like if you had a healthy relationship with food?

4. What would be different in your life if you had more energy, more mental clarity, and maintained your perfect weight?

CHAPTER II

WHY WE EAT

"Growth is painful. Change is painful. But nothing is as painful as staying stuck somewhere you don't belong."

—N. R. Narayana

INTRODUCTION

Here's a crazy question. Why does anybody eat? There's an obvious answer. You eat because you're hungry, or you eat to survive. There would be no need for this book in a perfect world where these are the only reasons.

The first step in your journey to free yourself from a toxic relationship with food is to ask that question. Most people, especially those singularly focused on one aspect of eating, their weight, often don't know the answer to that question.

In this chapter, let's explore some of my insights about why I was eating when I wasn't hungry and sometimes still do. I think it's helpful for you to identify the triggers that drive you to eat. This won't lead directly to taking control of your eating, but it's an important first step. The complete solution is coming.

But first of all, why do we eat?

PHYSICAL HUNGER

Many people are completely unaware of why they eat. Without giving it much thought, most people would automatically state that they eat because they're hungry. This is because they don't want to appear as if they're eating when they shouldn't. When I started examining why I was eating, I identified three different kinds of hunger. I'd say I was really hungry (in my stomach), I'm emotionally hungry (I just want to eat), or I'm 'mouth hungry' (I want to taste something).

Our bodies are wired to experience legitimate, real physical hunger. This chemical and physiological reaction happens in our brains and digestive systems to help us survive as individuals, society, and a species. All things would be equal if everyone operated as Mother Nature planned. Everyone would eat when they're hungry and stop when they're satisfied, which is quite a while before being full.

I don't believe many people operate this way 100% of the time. Despite having a wonderful relationship with food, I often miss the 'satisfied' signal and sometimes eat to the point of being too full. It's a logical conclusion then that if you don't properly listen to your body's built-in hunger gauge, you must be eating for other reasons.

ANXIETY/STRESS

The definition of anxiety is:

- a feeling of worry, nervousness or unease typically about an imminent event or something with an uncertain outcome.

(Oxford English Dictionary)

'An imminent event with an uncertain outcome' is something that's out of your control. Again, I'm not a doctor, so I can't address why you may experience stress. But the reason I experience stress is that I'm a bit of a control freak. If I feel I don't have control of certain outcomes, it creates a high level of anxiety.

Let's take writing this book, for example. I'd committed to writing this about six weeks before getting started. During that time, I felt so anxious. The voice in my head was screaming, "You don't have time to write a good book!" After all, I was committing to writing this in several months. The last book I wrote 20 years ago took me two and a half years. I noticed that my stress levels elevated, and sleep and eating patterns were affected during those weeks leading up to getting started.

Interestingly, the anxiety subsided once I rolled up my sleeves and started writing. This is an example of stress caused by something uncertain because you don't or can't get into the action to address it.

Whatever brings on stress for you may be a trigger to eat. Why do people think that eating at that moment will fix anything? My layperson's explanation is that the dopamine release from eating eases stress. Again, this is from my own experience and not based on scientific research. Suppose I'm right. In that case, the dopamine release is short-lived and will likely lead to more unnecessary eating. In the end, it creates more problems than the original anxiety you were trying to suppress or address.

It makes more sense to ask yourself what you could do to make the situation less stressful. In my case, I could've chosen to do some research for the book before starting to write.

I could have gone for a bike ride, or I could have started a knitting project. But I developed a habit many years ago to go straight for the food. Once I realized that my control issues triggered stress and put me in a position to feel vulnerable, I could learn to look at my choices in a different way.

BOREDOM

I once had a therapist explain to me that 'Type A' personalities, like me, need to be busy and productive as it makes them feel alive. She said we all need to feel productive to feel alive. It's just that Type A's find it harder to have downtime. These personalities are wired to feel like their identity is attacked when they don't feel productive. When I'm not feeling productive, I'm bored. Sometimes when I'm bored, I eat.

For some people, boredom is like a blow to their identity, bringing up many other emotions. It's not just a matter of not knowing what to do with yourself. The reality is that for me being bored generates anxiety. I know that, to this day, when I feel bored, my knee-jerk reaction is to go to the refrigerator. The good news is that when I realize that the anxiety is actually boredom, there are many things I can do other than eat.

Disordered eaters can also be driven to eat when they're bored. This could be because of habit or looking for the dopamine rush. Or it could be that the foods are designed to fill the void of boredom.

SADNESS AND GRIEF (NOT CLINICAL DEPRESSION)

Most people do not accept that they should experience the full spectrum of emotions. When you feel sad, you're uncomfortable with the feeling. Also, subconsciously you may believe that you should be happy all the time. Sometimes, this belief in constant happiness can create an additional level of anxiety.

Sadness and grief are brought on by events that could range from minor, such as not making it to a friend's wedding, to traumatic, such as when somebody close to you passes away.

For some people, food can provide comfort during those times, while others completely lose their appetite. For most of my adult life, I didn't realize this, but now I know I was someone who would first lose my appetite. Then after some time (depending on the severity of the situation), my appetite would return, and I'd start automatically binging on junk food. I'd tell myself I was entitled to do this because of whatever terrible event I'd just experienced. I realize now that I was using food to numb the sadness, and I was punishing myself with bad food choices rather than comforting myself. The consequences of eating, such as physical discomfort and disappointment with myself, sometimes lasted longer than the sadness over the original event.

EMOTIONAL EATING TO COMFORT, DISTRACT OR NUMB

The first step to freedom from a toxic relationship with food and toward a healthy relationship comes when you can identify the emotion and identify which of these you're trying to accomplish:

- comfort
- distraction
- numbing

You can usually find something else that will healthily serve the purpose. Go out for a hike or a bike ride, play the piano, do a jigsaw puzzle, snuggle up with your dog, cat or horse. I choose my horses every time.

I embarked on a journey of horsemanship just after my sister died. Coincidentally, it was the same time I began my journey toward a healthy relationship with food. I attribute both of these gifts in my life to my sister's passing. It was essential to turn that tragedy into something that added value in my life and others' lives. Again, I realized the opportunity to reflect on previously demonstrated disordered eating and turn the situation into something more positive.

CELEBRATIONS AND SOCIAL EVENTS

Most people can make good food choices when they're by themselves. But if there's an event coming up, look out! When it's your birthday, your friend's baby shower, your significant other's promotion at work, Valentine's Day, an invitation to a friend's party, the food holidays from Halloween through New Year's Day, or about a thousand other excuses to celebrate, all bets are off. Why is cake a

> ### 💣 Warning:
>
> Could it be that, in the case of your birthday, you think you deserve to spoil yourself when in fact, choosing the cake turns out to be a punishment of sorts, in the long run?
>
> Be aware that what you think is a 'treat' may well be a punishment because of your toxic relationship with food.

requirement at any major celebration? More importantly, why do you feel compelled to eat it?

The answer to the first question is, "Damned if I know." The answer to the second question may be found in my previous discussion about emotional eating. It could be that you're not entirely comfortable in social settings, or you experience peer pressure ("come on, just have one"), and you use the food for comfort or distraction or to please somebody else.

How about when you're invited to someone's home, and they make dinner for you? Do you have a voice in your head telling you how rude it'd be if you didn't eat what they serve? To appease social mores, you decide to eat. If it's something you wouldn't usually choose to eat or something you know will negatively affect how you feel afterward, you may also have an emotional reaction. At the same time, your commitment to yourself, how you feel, and your relationship with food may suffer. The self-abuse, and sometimes self-doubt and even self-loathing is perpetuated.

The following chapters will explore these situations and how to handle them.

FATIGUE AND LOW ENERGY

There is another feeling that will often drive you to food. When you're experiencing fatigue that results from lack of a good night's sleep or doing too much physically, have you ever thought, "I just need some food or sugar for energy?" Lo and behold, you eat whatever you eat, and you don't feel more energized. If you eat sugary foods, you may get a very brief insulin boost, but it'll be short-lived, and the after-effects may even exaggerate the feelings of tiredness.

This is less 'emotional' eating and more of your body telling you that all systems are not ok. You may underestimate how much being tired is related to your appetite. You may find it hard to accept that what you need is sleep and not food. Chapter IV will discuss the other lifestyle elements that need to be addressed if you want to be genuinely healthy, realizing all the benefits of a healthy relationship with food, including easily maintaining a healthy weight.

SATISFY A CRAVING OR ADDICTION

In the many years before I started my journey to a completely healthy lifestyle, I was sure that food could talk, or was it just talking to me? I know you know what I mean. Did you ever have Häagen Dazs ice cream calling to you from the freezer? It would always say something like, "You know you want me. You know if you eat me now, I won't be talking to you tomorrow night. You can start your diet tomorrow. After all, it's Sunday, and Monday is a good day to start over again." How about that amazing chocolate cake that shouts at you, "I'm going to be stale if you don't eat me tonight, and you know how much you hate to throw away food."

Whoa, wait a minute. What the heck? Why were these urges so strong? Why were the messages so loud? Was the food really talking to me? If you'd asked me these questions during those years, I'd have told you the reason was my lack of willpower or discipline.

Have you ever had a conversation with someone addicted to drugs or alcohol? Their experiences are very similar. This is the nature of addiction. Yes, food addiction is real. I used to say I wish I were a drug addict or an alcoholic. I figured I could solve my problem by eliminating those things from my life completely. From my experiences with anorexia, I found out that I couldn't just eliminate food from my life as much as I wanted to.

This was why I never believed I'd be normal around food. I'd decided to dig deep and find the discipline and will-power to manage my relationship with food and my decisions about when and what I was eating. I had to avoid getting to the point where I disgusted myself by a number on the scale or curled up into a ball of anxiety if I needed to go clothes shopping. That was the best I could do.

Addiction to certain foods is real. I'll discuss this in more detail in Chapter IV. One thing I'll tell you now is, rest assured, this isn't an addiction that willpower will cure.

HABITUAL OR RITUALISTIC EATING

Sometimes you may make certain food choices because it's a habit. This often goes hand-in-hand with 'traditional' food choices and tastes you develop when you're young. For example, my husband was raised by his French parents. There was wine with dinner every night and bread and cheese after dinner. When we first met, this was how he ate. It took many discussions, but I finally convinced him that there was no need to have bread and cheese every night after a full meal. He gave up the cheese, but there was still bread on the table with every meal.

Often, you don't think about what makes sense. You just do it because you always did it that way. The only way to break a habit is to stop doing it. It does get easier if you replace one habit with another. For example, remove the bread and cheese and put a fruit bowl out to end the meal. Voilà, a new habit is formed.

FOR THE TASTE

Earlier I discussed how there are foods that you may eat for comfort, not because your mouth likes the taste, but these are the foods that you've associated with good feelings when you were young. It's another kind of habitual eating. My girlfriend shared that she was raised with a 'salad' that consisted of a Jello mold with pineapple chunks and marshmallows. To this day, when she gets together with extended family, tasting this food is a must, even though it's something she'd not make for herself.

FOOD IS A TERRIBLE THING TO WASTE

Somehow one message that rang loud and clear throughout my childhood was that it was a crime to throw away food. I come from generations whose parents said, "Do

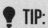 **TIP:**

When you have a healthy relationship with food, you can identify *why* you want to eat. Then, you can choose *what* you want to eat. Do you want to eat, or do you want to do something else that will soothe comfort or distract you?

Suppose you choose to eat for reasons other than hunger. In that case, eat foods that do not negatively impact you physically, mentally, emotionally or challenge and derail the relationship you worked so hard to create.

you know how many starving children there are in the world? How dare you leave food on your plate?" Intellectually you know that overeating or eating food that isn't good for you rather than throwing it away won't help those starving children. However, the message came over loud and clear and throwing food away or leaving it on your plate seemed to be a terrible thing to do. At some point, you must question the logic of some of your reasons for eating.

WHAT'S NEXT

The point of this chapter was to bring mindfulness into the discussion about the relationship you have with food. There are two elements to this relationship. One is why you eat, and the other is what you eat.

If you picked up this book because you've previously bought and read your fair share of diet books, you're sure to identify with Chapter III. It'll soon become clear why all that dieting rarely resulted in the long-term results you were seeking. If you still don't feel you have control over what you eat, what you weigh, or how you feel, this next chapter will explain why.

> "If you take responsibility for yourself, you will develop a hunger to accomplish your dreams."
>
> —Les Brown

CHAPTER II EXERCISE:

If you've never identified why you eat, what emotion is triggering you or what craving you're having, it'd be very helpful to do this exercise.

Personally, I take issue with 'diets' or nutritionists who would suggest you need to journal every calorie you eat and the feelings you have when you're eating. I don't believe this is sustainable. However, if you can identify the frequent recurring emotions and circumstances that drive you to eat, it may give you more transparency to an open, honest relationship with food.

1. The last time you ate mindlessly, or when you weren't hungry, what were you feeling? Was there an event that triggered that emotion?

2. If boredom triggers you to eat, figure out why boredom is an issue. What does being bored mean to you and your ego?

3. What activities do you enjoy doing that would be a better distraction than eating?

4. If you crave certain foods when you're not hungry, what foods do you crave?

CHAPTER III

THE FOUR-LETTER D-WORD (DIET)

"Sometimes it's hard to see the rainbow when there've been endless days of rain."

—Christina Greer

INTRODUCTION

The word 'diet' has become so loaded with emotion that it can be like a swear word to some people. The two definitions of 'diet' are:

- the kinds of food that a person, animal or community habitually eats (e.g., a vegetarian diet)
- a special course of food to which one restricts oneself, either to lose weight or for medical reasons (e.g., "I'm going on a diet")

(Oxford English Dictionary)

I'd argue that the order should be reversed in society today. To most people, the word diet implies doing something punitive, restrictive, or unpleasant.

It's time we expose the billion-dollar diet industry as one that gives you false hope and convinces you that you'll finally be thin if you just have enough willpower and follow the latest diet. By the way, they don't tell you at what expense. After reading this chapter, you'll be convinced never to try 'dieting' again.

DIETS ARE A TEMPORARY CHANGE

Many people who have gone through years of yoyo dieting have probably spent enough money on diet books, special foods, and special cookbooks to pay for at least one semester of tuition at the most elite schools. In retrospect, do you feel that money may have been better spent elsewhere?

Everywhere we look, there are new fads and new diets that are trending. This is why I'm committed to not, and have no interest in, writing a diet book.

It's also why I don't discuss how I eat or the foods I choose using the word 'diet.' Instead, if anyone asks me, I'm proud to say, "I follow a WFPB lifestyle," or "I choose to eat whole, plant-based foods," or "I'm a vegan." I'll discuss the distinct difference between a vegan lifestyle and a WFPB lifestyle in Chapter VI.

Many people have tried some sort of prescribed diet to lose weight. What have we learned from diets? They don't work. If they did, it wouldn't be a multi-billion dollar business. We'd go on a diet, and we'd be fixed.

Think about it. If you change something temporarily, why would you think that reverting to how you originally did that thing wouldn't undo the change you worked so hard to achieve? If you train to become a top athlete and stop training for a year, are you going to be able to participate in your sport at the level you were when you stopped training? Why would changing how you eat for a short time make a permanent change?

DIETS ARE ABOUT DEPRIVATION

Think about the smoker that wants to quit smoking. They'll often stop on a particular day or after they smoke this last pack. When they plan to quit, they stress over it and often 'binge smoke' leading up to that day. Even before that day arrives, there's a lot of anxiety because they know they must face the consequences of giving up a habit that has physically and psychologically served them. Giving up smoking will deprive them of the nicotine drug and the oral fixation that has been the smoker's habit for a long time.

Many people approach 'going on a diet' the same way. They're going to start Monday. So what do they do on the weekend before that Monday? They eat all the foods they think they'll struggle to give up for the particular diet, and they usually eat lots of them. As discussed in the previous chapter regarding emotional eating, there is anxiety in anticipating the deprivation that's to follow until you lose weight. You often use that as a 'pass' to eat whatever you want, often in large quantities. In my experience, and I'll bet for many others, the love-hate relationship with food rages all weekend. By Sunday night, you're looking forward to Monday, so you can stop abusing yourself, and for the fantasy that "this time I'm going to do it."

DIETS MEAN CONSTANT COUNTING

Most diets focus on counting calories or carbohydrates. There's very little focus on the overall complete nutrition of the foods. If you count calories, your brain spends time adding numbers that do not consider nutrition or health. It has you focusing on the quantity of food you can eat. Or, in reality, the quantity of food you're *forbidden* from eating. How's that for always feeling deprived?

Diets that focus on counting carbohydrates leave most people extremely deficient in specific nutrients. They often include eating high amounts of unhealthy, saturated fats. And while these diets allow for lots of low-carb, high-fat foods and plenty of calories, you're still depriving yourself of many foods you have been eating and craving. You may also be risking health issues.

DIETS MEAN WATCHING THE CLOCK

There is one other theme in the world of popular fad diets. These diets force you to decide what foods you'll eat based on the clock. One example is Intermittent Fasting (IF). While all the discussions about the advantages of IF are about how this affects your metabolism, many people think this is a way to lose weight regardless of the foods they eat and their relationship with food. The thinking is if I deprive myself of food for a certain number of hours, I'm free to eat whatever I want when I *do* eat. Wrong.

Another diet was written about years ago, suggesting you eat only fruit in the morning and nothing else. Other similar diets say that fruit should always be eaten before other foods, and they tout other specifics about the importance of eating food in a particular order. Again, I'm not convinced that any of this will do anything for you if the rest of what you eat isn't healthy.

I don't think anyone should be looking at the clock to determine when it's ok to eat. I also do not believe that, in the absence of a healthy relationship with the right foods, this has the potential to be any more effective than any other diet.

INTUITIVE EATING

Another hot topic in the world of fad diets is intuitive eating. Philosophically, intuitive eating suggests that nature built your body to tell you when you're hungry or satisfied and what foods or nutrients your body is craving. You just need to 'listen.' I'm sure if these ideas were trending at the start of my dieting life, I'd have tried it for about two days, insisting that my body was telling me that I needed French fries and chocolate bars. Today, I understand and can relate to intuitive eating, but earlier in my journey, no way!

KETO AND PALEO DIETS

The two most popular diets trending these days are Keto and Paleo diets. The Keto diet emphasizes a low carbohydrate, high protein, and high fat intake. Many people report successfully losing weight and feeling great, at least for the first few months they switch from the SAD. In the long term, however, there are concerns of high cholesterol, heart disease, and other issues (discussed further in Chapter V) with a high intake of animal proteins.

The Paleo diet supposedly focuses on lean meats, fish, vegetables, nuts and seeds that our ancestors consumed as hunter-gatherers. This diet removes all grains, dairy products and legumes. These foods are considered inflammatory by professionals who support this diet. There are some downsides to the Paleo diet, but, as mentioned in the Resources section, this is the basis of how Dr. Mark Hyman recommends his patients eat. Following this diet, his patients have achieved great improvement in their health.

However, the focus of this book is the path we choose to change our toxic relationship with food to a healthy one. Neither Keto nor Paleo was a path that would work for me.

SUPPLEMENTS TO HELP YOU DIET

Supplements have a place in your diet. However, do not fall for supplements that say they'll help you lose weight without changing anything else about what you eat. Some ads claim these products will melt fat, increase your metabolism, reduce your appetite or digest your food more efficiently. If you don't change what you eat, these things won't help weight loss, energy levels or overall health. There are few controls in the supplement industry. It's not unusual for somebody to slap a label on a bottle of pills and market it to those most vulnerable and most desperate for a solution. In many cases, this is worse than most fad diets.

IT SOUNDS LIKE INSANITY AFTER AWHILE

Isn't the definition of insanity doing the same thing repeatedly and expecting a different outcome? Many people are so fooled into believing that this time, this diet, this effort will be different. Many who have been on diets that don't work think there must be something wrong with them. They believe that they do not have the willpower to eliminate 'fattening foods.' They still believe it's about discipline. It's not.

Through the power of clever marketing, we've continued to fall for another diet by another name. I'm here to tell you, it's not about willpower, and it's not your fault.

Big food companies market their processed, diet foods (i.e., low calorie, low carbohydrate, etc.) to make us

> The food industry does not want you to know this, but they process many packaged foods in a way that makes them addictive. After all, what better way to guarantee a continuous source of revenue than to have you become addicted. Does this remind you of cigarettes?

believe they're good for us. Most packaged foods are so processed that whatever nutrition is left is minimal, compared to the harm they cause. What's worse is, if they're sold to us as a 'diet' or low-calorie food, implying or stating they'll help us lose weight, this may be true for the short time that you continue to restrict yourself just to eat those foods.

It's this feeling that you should have the willpower to be thin that derails your relationship with food. This will become clearer as I discuss nutrition in Chapter IV.

> Diets fail because they are focused strictly on weight loss, and they're not designed with a long-term health-oriented goal. The problem is not a lack of willpower. Diets are often not designed to feed us as nature intended.

KEEP IN MIND THE END GAME

There's a lot of lip service to 'loving oneself.' If you're practicing self-love, you're taking care of yourself. When you go on many of these prescribed diets, the goal is to lose weight. When you develop a healthy relationship with food, there is integrity in that love and self-care.

Diets emphasize losing weight with very little regard for being healthy. I feel confident stating that if you lose weight because you discover and create a healthy relationship with food, you'll have your health, vitality and maintain the weight you should be.

If you have weight to lose, and you endeavor to clean up your relationship with food forever, you'll lose the weight, but you'll also embrace the role that food plays in your life. You'll have the energy to play with your children and your grandchildren. You'll stave off the diseases that seem to run in your family. And you'll sleep better at night.

CHANGING YOUR RELATIONSHIP WITH FOOD IS DIFFERENT

Again, I reiterate, this is *not* another diet book. This is about creating a loving relationship with food and taking care of your health. Yes, I'll share some steps to success and suggestions on addressing your relationship with food *and* your health, but this will be a lifestyle change, not a temporary set of rules to follow and achieve a certain weight.

WHAT'S NEXT

Are you starting to feel better about yourself? Those diets that you tried that were gratifying for a short period were never meant to provide a long-term solution. Are you ready to start understanding how you're meant to eat?

It helps if you learn the basics of nutrition and how food nourishes and nurtures us. Chapter IV examines the basics of nutrition and the human body's wonderful, complex, and intricate systems. You're about to learn everything you need to know about reaching and maintaining your correct weight. This part of the book asks you to move forward in good faith and start addressing your relationship with food as a health issue and not a weight loss plan.

> *"The toughest part of a diet is not watching what you eat. It's watching what other people eat."*
>
> —Unknown

CHAPTER III EXERCISE:

If you've tried many diets in the past, it will be valuable to reflect on those experiences.

1. What motivated you to go on a diet at the time?

2. Why did you choose the specific diet that you chose?

3. If you feel these diets were unsuccessful, do you recall why? Did you feel deprived?

    a. Did you have difficulty overcoming cravings?

    b. Did you fail due to the environment, the wrong foods were in your house, or you attended events where you 'cheated?'

4. If you felt the diet was successful, what are you looking for now?

CHAPTER IV

NUTRITION

"The doctor of the future will no longer treat the human frame with drugs, but rather will cure and prevent disease with nutrition."

—Thomas Edison

INTRODUCTION

I've talked about the reasons we eat in Chapter II. I know you're anxious to get to the punchline and find out how to change your relationship with food. But first, you must understand how your body uses food and why you crave the foods you do. In Chapters I and II, I mentioned that many people are often not making their food choices of their own free will.

My journey led me down a total 'nutrition geek' path. I wanted to understand what choices I'd made and why. In retrospect, I didn't understand much about macro and micronutrients before starting this journey. I didn't understand how I metabolize what I eat. Most of what I did know, I likely learned from the mass marketing of the foods I was eating. Today, food is a wonderful part of my life. I still love to 'geek out' on the newest studies with insights into how I can use food to enhance my quality of life, give me pleasure in experiencing wonderful flavors and experiences, and keep me healthy.

I realize that there is only so much that you, the reader, can digest at one time. I also realize that not everyone likes to know about every study and detail of how human bodies use food. Therefore, I share basic information to help you understand why your journey should follow a certain path. If you want to research any of these topics further, I offer many sources that I learned from in the Resources section at the end of the book.

CLEAN EATING

What is clean eating? When I discuss clean eating, I'm referring to eating whole foods that aren't processed. That means no additives that act as preservatives or flavor enhancers. A Whole-Food (WF) food plan would include lots of fruits, vegetables, whole grains, lean (ideally plant) proteins, and healthy fats. Generally, this refers to staying around the perimeter of your grocery store.

Whole clean foods are becoming prevalent in the freezer section as well. Farms realize that they can leave out the preservatives if they flash-freeze fruits, vegetables, and wholegrain bread (no, not ice cream). Flash-frozen produce is often more nutrient-dense than the same items you'd purchase from the produce section. Those items in the produce department may have been off the plant for several days. They may also sit in your refrigerator for days after purchase. Nutrients in all plants diminish once they're picked.

ADDICTION (SPECIFICALLY TO FOOD)

PSYCHOLOGICAL ADDICTION

The definition of addiction is:

- a compulsive need for and use of a habit-forming substance. It's accepted as a mental illness in the diagnostic nomenclature and results in substantial health, social and economic problems.

(National Institute on Drug Abuse)

There has been much research on this topic, particularly in light of the current opioid addiction epidemic in the US.

Johann Hari's work, *Chasing the Scream: The First and Last Days of the War on Drugs*, focuses on the relationship between addiction and social connection. His research shows a higher risk of substance addiction when there is no connection with loved ones, peers and others.

Gabor Mate, MD, published a book, *In the Realm of Hungry Ghosts*, and a documentary film. Both look at the connection between trauma (usually experienced as a child) and substance addiction as an adult.

Anna Lembke, MD, focuses on the neuroscience of addiction in her book, *Dopamine Nation: Finding Balance in the Age of Indulgence*. Her research reveals that even with supportive friends and family and without trauma, there is still the possibility of addiction. She explains how the chemical reaction in the brain and release of high levels of dopamine feeds addictive behavior. Addicts will continue to seek out whatever it is that creates the dopamine release.

When dealing with my eating disorders, food addiction wasn't taken seriously. Even today, when you say someone is an addict, you're usually referring to substance or alcohol abuse. Or perhaps you're talking about sex or gambling addicts. But, if you have a healthy relationship with food, it's hard to imagine unhealthy food addiction as a problem.

From my personal experience, I believe the explanations for addiction above are true. But, I think Dr. Lembke's explanation makes the most sense, especially to those addicted to the dopamine rush food provides. Also, Dr. Lembke's explanation gives us full responsibility for our behavior without blaming the environment in which we were raised.

CHEMICAL ADDICTION

Perhaps the large food companies don't want to acknowledge there's such a thing as unhealthy food addiction. It's just like the tobacco companies who didn't want to acknowledge that cigarettes were addictive. The good news is that recently there has been more focus on addictions to specific foods. Therefore, it's appropriate that you identify and understand that some of your poor relationships with food center on an addiction problem.

Remember in Chapter II when you looked at eating to numb you from feeling negative emotions? What better way to avoid feeling bad than identifying immediate gratification? Or chasing a lift from a good dose of dopamine? Food addiction has two components. One is the behavior of using food to numb negative emotions. The other is the chemical addiction created in the kitchens of large food companies.

It's now known that food companies use additives in their food designed to create an addiction. There is a term for this. Many people become addicted to 'hedonic eating.'

Hedonic eating is defined as:

- A preoccupation with and desire to consume foods for the purposes of pleasure and in the absence of physical hunger.

(Oxford English Dictionary)

This directly results from the additives and refined (processed) ingredients in our food supply. Remember the Lay's Potato chips commercial with the tagline, "Betcha can't eat just one?" That was more than a catchy slogan. It was a challenge to defy what the formula was made to accomplish!

Eating foods you enjoy provides a dopamine release. Being addicted to eating certain unhealthy foods is a function of the 'normal' dopamine release and your body's physiological response to processed foods. You're fighting a double whammy when you eat addictive, processed foods.

THE MICROBIOME

In Chapter II, you looked at the behavioral side of your food addictions, such as eating by habit as a reaction to your emotional state. In this chapter, I've introduced psychological and chemical addiction. Now, let's look at the digestive process to understand this chemical addiction to certain foods.

It's widely accepted that when you eat addictive foods, such as sugar, your brain is triggered to drive you back to the same foods. This is only partially true. Research[5] shows that much more is happening, and it originates in the microbiome.

The microbiome is all the bacteria in your intestinal tract. It has a lot more responsibility regarding your health than you probably realized. It's where all the good and bad bacteria that aid your digestion lives. It's also now believed to be the root of the addictive drive to eat certain foods continually.

A simple way of looking at this is that the good bacteria do their job properly processing nutrients from your food. They slough off the waste (our poop) and hopefully some bad bacteria. If you have lots of bad bacteria, the good bacteria can't do their job well. Also, the bad bacteria can damage the lining of your intestinal tract and interfere with the proper digestion of your food. This explains why many people often suffer from constipation and irregular bowel movements.

The bad bacteria can perforate the lining of the intestine. When this happens, the bacteria leak out of your intestinal tract into the rest of your body. This can be very dangerous and is now thought to increase the risk of cancer and other chronic diseases.

Consuming foods high in fiber is important for your digestive system to operate properly. Unfortunately, the SAD has low amounts of fiber. Fermented foods are also good for your digestion. While fiber keeps things working well, fermented foods add diversity. The more diverse the bacteria in your microbiome, the better.

These bacteria are very influential in your overall health. If you have many bad bacteria, fewer healthy white blood cells are produced. This affects your overall immune system. The opposite is true too. If you eat clean, healthy foods without additives, preservatives, or processed (foreign) ingredients, you'll have a stronger immune system. You'll also have more regular, healthier bowel movements.

FOOD ADDICTION IS CAUSED BY THE FOOD YOU EAT

The other thing that happens with the bacteria in your gut is that, as living organisms, they have a survival mechanism. If the bad bacteria results from eating sugar, for example, it's actually in its best interest that you continue to feed it sugar for its survival.

Your microbiome has a direct connection to your brain. When the bad bacteria start taking over, that connection is overrun with messages of 'more, more, more,' which you'll feel as cravings. The bad bacteria wants to build up its army. The only way to do that is to constantly send out recruiting messages in the form of very strong cravings and get the host (you) addicted. In the sugar example, the cravings will be specifically for the processed sugar you find in candy, sodas, pastries and many processed foods. An addiction is born. Keep in mind that the example cites sugar because most people can relate to that. The same thing happens with so many additives in processed foods. The more you eat, the more you crave.

Some of the most addictive foods are processed sugar, and wait for it, cheese. Yes, cheese! I think most people have experienced the addictive nature of sugar. But many people have no idea that cheese is an addictive food. Most people grew up thinking that milk and dairy were good for us. I'll discuss this further in Chapter VI. I can only shock your whole belief system so much at a time without fearing I'll lose you.

With a belief system that milk is good for humans, many people assume that cheese must be good for them too. In fact, casein, a component of all dairy products and particularly concentrated in cheese, releases an opiate when digested called casomorphins. Therefore, eating cheese creates both a psychological and physiological addiction. This is in addition to the inflammatory reaction created by all dairy products.

The bottom line is this. Food addiction is real, whether generated by the dopamine surge or the bad bacteria's drive to survive and multiply. The only way to break the cycle is to remove those foods from your system. Then, find out if you're somebody who can reintroduce these foods in small amounts without getting cravings (more on this in the next chapter).

OUR POOR TASTE BUDS

But wait, it gets better. In addition to feeling out-of-control cravings, many people have deadened taste buds. This keeps the cycle of 'more, more, more' going. It's terrible for your health and likely your weight. Most people who eat a SAD feel the need to add more sugar to sweet foods and salt to other foods.

HORMONE IMBALANCE

I've already discussed the impact on the microbiome when you eat unhealthy, processed foods. Processed foods create chaos and wreak havoc throughout your body. Another problem caused by this is hormone imbalance.

Hormones control functions in your body, such as reproductive, metabolic, and more. Many of these hormones work in harmony with each other. I'm not just talking about male and female reproductive hormones. Hormones have far more diversity than just controlling reproduction.

I do not intend to provide a scientific explanation of how hormones work, as the endocrine systems are integrated and therefore complex. It's only my intention to share with you that if you're struggling with weight, health or chronic fatigue, you should request hormone functioning tests from your doctor.

Here are some of the hormones that your doctor should discuss with you:

- T3 and T4 are hormones that control your thyroid activity. Your thyroid regulates your metabolism. Your metabolism is the rate at which you burn calories and regulate how your body uses the nutrients for fuel.
- Cortisol is often called the stress hormone, and it keeps you safe. It kicks in to respond to fight or flight (survival reaction) in a stressful situation.
- Insulin is a very important hormone. When you eat healthy carbohydrates, they're broken down and stored as glucose. This is the body's main source of energy. Insulin regulates the levels of blood glucose through your circulatory system.
- Melatonin and serotonin control your sleep and your moods.
- Dopamine is the pleasure hormone.
- Reproductive hormones, such as estrogen, progesterone and testosterone, help develop and maintain gender characteristics. When they aren't balanced, they can cause issues with fertility and even hormone-related cancers.

Finally, there are other hormones in your body that many people don't think about often, and unfortunately, rarely does their family doctor. An example is DHEA, which is produced in the adrenal glands and helps your body produce some of the other hormones mentioned above. For this reason, my recommendation is that you go to a professional who understands integrative and functional medicine. They will look at how well your whole body works together.

What happens when any or all of your hormones are out of balance? That's like asking what happens when you blow out a tire or run out of gas in your car. Like a car, your body is an integrated system of parts (organs). If a part is faulty, then the whole machine runs inefficiently at best, or worse, not at all. You know what that looks like in a car, but do you miss the signs in your body?

SYMPTOMS OF MACHINE BREAKDOWN

While I discussed the microbiome and hormones separately, keep in mind that they work together. It's just like a car's carburetor and pistons. I'm showing my age here as cars no longer have carburetors! When there is a hormone imbalance or a microbiome imbalance, your whole system works inefficiently. Just like the signals you get when your car's engine needs attention (i.e., noises, dashboard indicators, inability to accelerate), you may often ignore signs and signals from your body.

One of the most common symptoms is fatigue. Sometimes the fatigue is chronic regardless of how much sleep you get. Sometimes it's due to insomnia or other sleep disorders (often the result of a hormonal or nutritional imbalance). You may also struggle from brain fog and the inability to focus or maintain mental clarity.

> ### ☄ Warning:
>
> Don't automatically blame your metabolism for weight gain. You must look at what you're eating and your relationship with food. Your metabolism may be faulty, causing you to gain or lose weight when you don't want to. However, most people use their metabolism as an excuse for weight gain. The reality is they're victims of food addictions and have a diet of unhealthy, processed foods.

Recent studies[6] have shown that the metabolic rate does not decrease with age until around 60. Even then, it's only about 1% per year. However, people tend to gain weight with age because their activity level decreases. They tend to eat more and burn less.

Another symptom may be the irregularity of your bowel movements. I can't talk about food intake without telling you that you should at least take a peek at your poop. Chronic diarrhea or constipation is such a widespread problem amongst women that many believe it is 'normal.' It's not. Too often, many people use over-the-counter laxatives. This is like putting a Band-Aid on an infected wound and offering no other treatment.

I had many of the above symptoms. However, the overwhelming problem was chronic fatigue that progressed over several years. That was the final straw. It was debilitating and impacted day-to-day life. It motivated me to finally free myself from my toxic relationship with food and start my journey to the healthy relationship I have with food today. I didn't even think about whether I'd lose weight. I just wanted my energy back. Weight loss, mental clarity and regular bowel movements were added benefits.

INFLAMMATION

Inflammation is the immune system's automatic response when something isn't right in your body. This could be an injury. It also happens when you introduce a foreign substance to your body. The inflammation is the blood going to that area to fix the problem. In the case of injury, it adds padding and protection to the injured area.

Inflammation from food is an allergic reaction. It can range from minor to life-threatening. Food allergy incidents have increased dramatically in the past 25 years. This is due to the chemicals widely used in our conventional (non-organic) food supply. When you eat processed foods, you introduce unnatural, foreign substances into your body. Your body reacts. Processed sugar and dairy are two of the most common inflammatory foods in the SAD.

If you get out of bed feeling bloated or achy (without any other activity-related explanation), it's almost certainly due to your diet. This chronic inflammation also impacts your mental state, including mental clarity, mood swings, and even dementia and Alzheimer's.

Before my food changes, I had many orthopedic injuries. My system couldn't tolerate non-steroidal anti-inflammatory drugs (NSAIDs) like aspirin or ibuprofen. Therefore, I struggled with inflammation. I assumed it was because of past injuries and arthritis. I had my first of three back surgeries while still eating a SAD. As I wasn't a fan of narcotics, my recovery was slow and painful.

> The truth is you don't know how much you suffer from inflammation until it's not there.

I'd dropped gluten, artificial sweeteners, and most processed foods by my second back surgery. I was shocked with how much easier my recovery was as compared to the first surgery. By the time I had my third back surgery three years ago, I was only eating WFPB foods. After five days in the hospital, I could walk up and down my street with very little pain. It was miraculous. There is no other reasonable explanation besides changing the foods I eat.

MACRO AND MICRONUTRIENTS

Macronutrients include protein, carbohydrates, and fats. Most people know we need them. However, most people don't know how much of each is needed. There is more to these nutrients than counting grams. All nutrients have specific jobs. They work together to promote energy, strength, growth, repair, and other processes. But like everything else in your body, they do not work alone. For example, in the absence of healthy fats, you can't digest and utilize the protein in your food.

Your body also requires many micronutrients (vitamins and minerals) to function well. It's hard to get the recommended daily requirement of micronutrients in the SAD of highly processed foods. There are healthy and unhealthy proteins, carbs and fats. If you eat unhealthy foods to get these nutrients, there is a negative impact on your overall health.

Bacon, for example, offers a complete protein and a portion of fats. But there are also carcinogens and quite a bit of cholesterol. So, you've got your protein, but there is a price to pay. Donuts offer you plenty of carbohydrates and fats. But, with the use of processed flour, sugar and deep-frying in highly processed oil, there isn't one valuable calorie left.

As discussed before, with all the processing in the above examples, your body experiences inflammation. You're creating significant imbalances hormonally and in your microbiome. Whatever nutrients were in the foods' raw ingredients are inaccessible for digestion.

NON-GMO AND ORGANIC?

If you want to eat healthy, clean foods, stay away from Genetically Modified Organisms (GMO) foods. These are foods where the DNA is altered. The use of glyphosates is a well-known example. Research[7] has shown that consuming GMO foods can compromise your immune system. Your immune system does not recognize it as something you should be eating. The way we're treat-ing our food supply contributes to the higher incidences of cancer, ADHD, autism and extreme food allergies in children.

I know many people think if they eat processed foods with organic ingredients, they're eating healthy. It's not the case. If the ingredients have been processed (i.e., heating, adding preservatives, etc.), the nutrients and your ability to digest them have been compromised. It doesn't matter if the processed foods are organic or not. However, if you eat whole foods that aren't processed, how important is eating organic? Because of the genetic engineering and chemicals that have been introduced into our food supply chain, it's becoming more important to consider organic foods whenever possible.

There are certain foods where it's more important to choose organic than others. These are fruits and vegetables exposed to pesticides and other chemicals with no protection (e.g., berries). On the other hand, I believe it's less critical to buy organic fruits and vegetables with thicker non-edible skins such as avocados.

It's easy to find support on this topic in many blogs, articles and research papers on the internet. One thing is certain. If you have a choice between eating a non-organic apple or a box of organic potato chips, go for the apple every time.

HYDRATION, HYDRATION, HYDRATION

Water is critical to all of our bodily functions. Many people do not realize that our bodies are made up of an average of 60% water. The percentage is slightly higher with men while a little lower with women. If we do not stay hydrated, our blood can't circulate properly, our digestive system is very inefficient, and basically, all of our organs are impacted. If we don't hydrate properly, we will experience any or all of the following: fatigue, dizziness, headaches, constipation. Overall, physical and mental performance will be compromised.

If you are not accustomed to drinking lots of water throughout the day, you may not know how much you need. This will vary with activity level, heat exposure, weight and other factors. The guide that helps me identify if I am drinking enough is the color of my pee. You should be urinating fairly frequently, and it should be a very pale yellow. Anything darker, and you are taxing your bodily functions.

DEFINE HEALTHY

So how do you get the recommended amount of nutrients? The answer is, eat whole foods that haven't been processed. This gives your entire system the fuel it needs to run properly and efficiently.

However, there's more to being healthy than having a great relationship with food. As you start your journey to this healthier relationship, you'll want to pay attention to being the healthiest person you can be. It's time to look at the other critical elements your body needs.

- **Exercise.** Your body and mind are built to be active. You don't need to suddenly run a marathon (although you may want to soon), but you do need to be active.
- **Sleep.** Be sure to get enough sleep. Eight hours is the average for an adult, but you may find it's more or less for you.
- **Engage socially.** We're social animals, and a lot of research indicates a negative effect on us if we're isolated. It can affect both your mental and physical health. Stay socially engaged with people you feel you have things in common.
- **Engage mentally.** The brain acts in the same way as other muscles in your body. It'll atrophy much faster with age if you don't use it.

The bottom line is, if you eat well, sleep well, stay engaged both physically and mentally, manage your stress level and hang out with friends, then your life will be enriched. You're taking responsibility for your health, and you won't need to worry about your weight ever again.

WHICH IS MORE IMPORTANT, FOOD INTAKE OR ACTIVITY?

When I was focused on my weight, I assumed managing my ratio of caloric intake to calories burned was the secret to being thin. For me, that was great. I like to exercise. Therefore, I'd just exercise more. I exercised compulsively. Unfortunately, it wasn't the answer to losing weight, feeling stronger, or having a healthy relationship with food.

Suppose you want to be healthy, including maintaining your healthy weight. In that case, you're better off eating very healthy foods and exercising moderately. You won't get the results you want by doing extreme exercise and eating healthy foods just 70% of the time. Food intake trumps activity.

WHAT'S NEXT

Let's review what you've discovered. Your body works like a machine, with food as fuel. There are other elements of a healthy lifestyle besides eating healthily. If you want to have the best quality of life and minimize your risk of disease, it's up to you to take responsibility for your health.

Are you ready to experience freedom from a toxic relationship with food and get on the path to an amazing relationship?

I hope you're reading and digesting (pun intended) this book slowly. While there is no quick fix here, if you chew on all of the topics discussed, you'll start seeing results in how you feel within a few short weeks. You may even see positive changes in your weight. Be patient with yourself and the process. You're starting a journey that will take you in the right direction for the rest of your life.

> *"If you think the pursuit of good health is expensive and time-consuming, try illness."*
>
> —Lee Swanson

CHAPTER IV EXERCISE:

In this chapter, you will have started to get an insight into what foods you've been eating that aren't working for you.

1. Identify those foods that you constantly overeat.

2. Do you often experience constipation or irregularity?

3. Identify the foods that make you feel bloated after eating them or the next day, or that may make you irregular.

4. What foods do you currently eat that you don't think you can give up?

    a. When do you eat these foods?

    b. Why would it be difficult to give these foods up?

CHAPTER V

LET THE JOURNEY BEGIN

"We often dismiss small changes because they don't seem to matter much in the moment."

—James Clear

INTRODUCTION

If you've been convinced through lots of trial and error that yoyo dieting won't work to keep you thin, sane, healthy, or improve your relationship with food, here is the roadmap for the journey that will do all of the above.

I'll talk about the importance of setting yourself up for success, from perusing the foods in your home to treating yourself kindly and making those good decisions regardless of where you are in your journey. Finally, be aware that your chances for success may depend on having a support system during the most challenging first weeks or months.

THIS IS YOUR JOURNEY — PROCEED WITH CONFIDENCE

You're ready to embark on your journey and make a huge lifestyle change. Good for you! I'm proud of you and want you to be proud of yourself. Unfortunately, you can't count on everyone around you being as supportive as you'd like. I want to share with you some obstacles you're likely to encounter.

You're going to get pushback from a lot of people. One of the phrases you'll hear is, "I eat healthily, I eat whatever I want, and I eat everything in moderation." You may even hear this from your doctor, as she prescribes medication for your high blood pressure and high cholesterol, antacids for your reflux, and laxatives for your constipation. In most cases, there are two problems with that statement. First, most people think the definition of moderation is "not all the time but whenever I want," or the other definition could be "not as much as I used to eat." Not very specific, is it? Second, how's that working out for them?

The pushback mostly comes from people who fought to feel better and maintain a healthy weight. However, they don't know how to do this and are afraid to try and fail at another diet. For many of those folks, resignation has set in. We all hit that point at some time in our journey. I know I did. Be kind to those people and stay committed to your journey. You can be the best teacher as a role model and not in heated debates trying to convince them.

DISCUSSIONS ALONG THE WAY

The time for discussion with these naysayers is when you're starting to make progress in your journey. I've noticed that if someone loses a tremendous amount of weight, they get asked how they did it. If the explanation is some diet or other, often those asking become interested and consider trying that diet. As discussed in Chapter III, this is rarely a long-term solution to weight loss or better health.

However, I've also noticed that when I explain to people that my health and energy are significantly better than before adopting a WFPB lifestyle, I rarely get asked how I did it. Too often, the immediate knee-jerk reaction is, "Oh, I could never do that," or "I could never give up (whatever their favorite junk food is)."

Again, share gently, and appreciate that this is a journey you're taking for yourself. Do not let these comments dissuade you.

ONE STEP AT A TIME TO CLEAN EATING

I discussed 'clean eating' in Chapter IV. Because this is the secret to a healthy relationship with food, I want to reiterate the meaning of clean eating.

> Clean eating is eating whole foods that aren't processed. Clean eating is the secret to success for better health, weight loss, and a healthy relationship with food.

Let's get started on your journey.

By now, you've probably been wondering how and why this is different from dieting. I'm glad you asked. I'm going to ask you to be open-minded throughout this chapter.

I'm going to ask you to change what you eat, one food group at a time. This will include the different food groups that aren't consistent with clean eating. As soon as there is an adjustment in your microbiome, taste buds and eating

> To realize freedom from a toxic relationship with food, you'll need to make changes to what you eat for the rest of your life. Rather than eliminating foods temporarily to lose weight, you will be eliminating foods that are putting toxins in your body that compromise your weight and your health!

habits, you'll start noticing that this isn't a struggle. It takes four to six weeks to adjust cravings and habits formed around eating. On your journey, if you select one food group at a time and find appropriate substitutions for those first four to six weeks, you'll be rewarded with losing the desire for that food as well as feeling better. All that without the feeling of deprivation, at least not for very long.

As the journey progresses, you'll forget how difficult it was to give up these foods if you're true to yourself. In many cases, even if you previously felt you couldn't live without these foods, chances are you'll completely lose interest in them. As you reduce the unhealthy foods that you eat, you'll find an abundance of other, healthier foods to take the place of the unhealthy foods.

SEE A DOCTOR AND GET A BASELINE BEFORE YOU START

Before starting your journey, get a referral to a doctor who practices functional medicine (or integrated medicine, as it's often referred to). Get this doctor to run tests to measure hormones, complete blood panel, inflammation, cholesterol, etc. These tests are useful to determine what improvements you'll see with better food choices. They're also useful to determine if you need to take any supplements. All vegans should be taking B12 supplements, and most people require other supplements (i.e., vitamin D, zinc, magnesium, to name a few) regardless of what they eat. Most internists and GPs do not do thorough testing nor understand how to interpret the results of standard blood tests. Doctors who practice functional medicine are better educated in nutrition and using food to treat us. I get my blood work done every six to nine months. It helps me determine any adjustments to supplements that I take.

ONE FOOD GROUP AT A TIME

My journey started with dipping my toe in the water ten years ago. I eliminated one food group at a time. The key to success was to find a good substitution for the thing I was eliminating. To select an appropriate substitution, identify the food and why you want to eat it. I'll take you through my journey of the foods I eliminated, and I'll share with you what worked as a substitution for the challenging first days or weeks of each change. You may opt to group the unhealthy foods differently than I did. Or you could choose to eliminate them in a different order. This is absolutely fine so long as you follow through and eliminate foods that aren't 'clean' from your diet.

 TIP:

When the going gets tough, review your list of objectives from the Chapter I Exercise. Then look in the mirror, and ask yourself, "Am I worth it?" Remind yourself this is self-love. This is what it looks like to take care of yourself. Find something healthy to eat, or do something other than eating.

ARTIFICIAL SWEETENERS

Before beginning my journey, I'd have told anyone who asked that I eat healthily. The one 'vice' was my diet soda, which I'd been addicted to since the age of 16. For 45 years, diet soda offered a sweet treat and kept me pumped up on caffeine for hours without adding any calories to my day. By my 20s, I had a six-pack-a-day diet soda habit (or was it an addiction?) This was after my morning coffee with four packs of the latest 'perfectly safe for you' artificial sweetener, the last one being aspartame.

I decided it was time to address this 40-year habit and start my journey by eliminating the artificial sweeteners. Given I consumed much more artificially sweetened products than those sweetened with sugar, I was shocked at the changes I felt within a week or two. I quickly noticed that any sweetened foods, including my one-cup-per-morning coffee with aspartame, suddenly tasted too sweet.

At the beginning of my journey, this stuck out in my mind, with no idea where it would lead me. The hardest part of eliminating artificial sweeteners was the concern that I'd gain weight if I eliminated all these zero-calorie foods and beverages. Also, before taking that first step, I anticipated feeling the same 'diet deprivation' that I'd experienced so many times before. I also believed that I'd always crave sweet foods. I couldn't imagine a day when that wouldn't be the case. That day did come, and it didn't take all that long. For me the elimination of artificial sweeteners was a great start.

After cutting out my diet soda and artificial sweeteners, I realized two things after that first month. First, I didn't miss them, and second, my worst fears didn't come true. I didn't gain weight, and I'd no desire to substitute the previously consumed zero-calorie sweeteners with high-calorie processed sugary foods.

Armed with this shockingly simple and effective experience, I was excited. By then, I was still considering that these changes would make me feel better, and I trusted they wouldn't result in weight gain. Both were important goals for me. But certainly, I felt like I had my priorities in order.

A great substitution for artificially sweetened beverages is water with or without fruit, such as berries, lemon, watermelon, or whatever fruit you love. Another idea is sparkling water, plain or fruit-infused. Add cinnamon (this adds a sweet taste to anything) to coffee or tea. Or you can wean yourself onto unsweetened or less sweetened tea or coffee with honey or a drop of maple syrup.

GLUTEN

The next thing I eliminated from my diet was gluten. Why? Because I accidentally discovered that I didn't feel well when I ate gluten. As I said previously, my husband, Roger, was the primary food person for the years we raised our three sons. He made lots of pasta and served French bread with every meal.

Then, after all the kids were grown and out of the house, Roger's work had him living away from home during the week for several years. My weeknight dinner became a salad thrown together with everything I could find in the refrigerator. When my husband was home on weekends, we'd have our typical dinners again with lots of bread and pasta. I realized that I felt awful on Monday mornings, and by Friday, I felt much better.

Gluten is a protein found in wheat, rye, barley, and other grains. If someone has celiac disease, they're completely incapable of processing this protein. Many others find out that they're gluten intolerant. There are long and short-term health implications for anyone who is gluten intolerant and consuming these grains, but it's not as severe as the effects on celiac patients.

There are many schools of thought from the doctors who research the effects of gluten. Some say that everyone will become gluten intolerant if we eat enough of these grains. Others say that's not the case. The best way to know if you're gluten intolerant is to stop eating it for about four to six weeks and then reintroduce it back into your system.

After eliminating gluten from your diet, if you're intolerant, the symptoms will be exaggerated once it's reintroduced. For me, the symptoms were terrible cramping, bloating and systemic inflammation. Now more than ten years later, if I have so much as a hint of gluten, I'll know within several hours, and the pain can be quite severe. The other problem for those that can't tolerate gluten is that it causes significant damage to your intestinal tract in the form of a 'leaky gut.' One meal with gluten can take weeks or months to get out of your system and allow your gut to recover.

I suggest you try to eliminate gluten for a full month at some point in your journey to find out if it's causing inflammation. If you find out you're gluten intolerant, elimination will show a tremendous improvement in how you feel. And if nothing changes, lucky you!

I promise you that I love bread and pasta as much as anyone I know. But suddenly, when I felt so much better after a meal, I had all the motivation I needed never to eat gluten-laden products again. I discovered Gluten-Free (GF) pasta made with beans, lentils and rice flour. All are high in protein and taste great. There are even a few GF bread types that I love. But if I can't get those specific bread types, it doesn't matter as I do not miss bread.

Substitutions include GF pasta made with only beans, lentils, rice, or other GF grains (without additives) and GF bread (stay away from the commercially available ones if they're highly processed). I found a couple of different ones I love at our local farmer's market. I bake my own using a few simple oat bread recipes when I can't get those. I make my own GF pizza crust. It's so easy and so good! I'm happy to share these recipes. Just contact me (details are in the Keep in Touch section at the back of the book). Use tamari instead of regular soy sauce, as gluten is in soy sauce. If you eat chocolate, check that it's GF. Many are not. Also, there are some good GF bagels available.

MILK DOES YOUR BODY GOOD — OR DOES IT?

Until recently, most moms feed their babies breast milk or formula until they're one year old. Then they transition their babies to drinking cow's milk like it's a rite of passage. There's lots of research[8] demonstrating that this isn't a good idea. Female mammals can reproduce and feed their babies from their mammary glands (breasts). Humans have babies and, ideally, feed them human breast milk. Likewise, cows are equipped to have babies and feed them cow's milk.

As a side note, I just bred my wonderful mare. As I witness the bonding between a mother and her baby, as she nurses, I'm again reminded how this is a baby's best chance at starting on a healthy journey through nutrition as nature intended. Would I think at any time to get cow's milk to feed my baby horse after I weaned her? Hell no. However, we're feeding our children milk from cows because that's the way we've always done it and because the dairy industry has convinced us that it's a good thing.

I'm convinced that this isn't what Mother Nature intended from the research I've reviewed. The milk from any mammal has the optimum nutrients to nourish the offspring of that species. Additionally, there are hormones in the milk of each of these mammals. The human body recognizes the hormones in cow's milk as a foreign body. I discussed in the previous chapter about the inflammation that happens when you introduce something your immune system thinks is an invader.

There has been more research with girls than boys into the effect of the hormones related to early puberty and cancer risk due to dairy consumption. As mentioned earlier, cheese is particularly bad because it's not only an inflammatory food, but it's also addictive due to casomorphins.

Dairy products were the next foods that I eliminated from my diet due to testing high for some of my gut's bad bacteria and chronic inflammation.

Substitutions include nut milk, oat milk, and soy milk. With these substitutions, please read the ingredients! Many are sweetened and processed with less than desirable ingredients.

Cheese substitutes are a little trickier as many dairy-free versions are highly processed with unhealthy fats and other ingredients. I've found a couple of clean, good brands. I'm happy to share my favorites if you reach out to me (details in the Keep in Touch section at the back of the book). Lots of recipes call for nutritional yeast as a great substitute for cheese. It has some health benefits and adds a cheesy flavor.

I sprinkle it on my healthy popcorn and use it in many pasta recipes. I no longer use sauce or cheese on pizza. I load my GF crust with lots of veggies. Sometimes instead of pizza sauce, I use a cheesy vegan sauce (i.e., pesto or alfredo) made with nutritional yeast, or a layer of mashed beans under the veggies, or just bake the pizza with veggies and drizzle (infused) balsamic vinegar on top. I don't miss a cheesy pizza at all, despite the fact it was one of my top five no-restraint foods when I didn't know better.

SUGAR

When I finally found a functional medicine doctor to work with me in diagnosing my extreme fatigue, my first reaction was relief. She believed me when I said, "I'm not crazy. My extreme chronic fatigue is not in my head." She started running tests to show that I had an abundance of bad bacteria (candida and others) in my gut and inflammation throughout my body. She suggested that I give up dairy and sugar for the next six weeks. Additionally, she gave me some very specific supplements for those six weeks. She explained that this was the only way to get the balance back in my microbiome.

Ironically, I owned a retail and wholesale frozen yogurt business at the time. I was often so busy running around during the day to our different locations that a cup of yogurt with nuts or fruit was all I ate. After ten minutes of whining to the doctor that I couldn't eliminate my frozen yogurt lunches, I had to admit I was still struggling with chronic fatigue. She assured me that her request was to eliminate this temporarily. After four to six weeks, I could decide what I wanted to do.

I went home and marked my calendar for four weeks. Sugar substitutes, sugar alcohols, honey, and syrup were not allowed to enter my body. I promise you, after two weeks of no sugar, no dairy, no yogurt, I started feeling so much better. I was starting to get some of my energy back. Each step and each food group eliminated made such a marked difference.

About six months earlier, I thought my inflammation was gone. It's all relative. Yes, I did feel better after I eliminated gluten, as the inflammation was reduced. I had no idea what it would feel like if I removed all inflammatory foods from my diet. Most people don't know what it feels like not to be chronically inflamed when they've always eaten the same way. Six weeks later, I returned to the doctor with a big smile on my face and a decision that I'd sell the yogurt business as soon as it made sense.

Substitutions for sugar include fruit, fruit and fruit. If I ever feel like I just want something sweet, I eat fruit. It's hard to overeat fruit, and it's so good for you containing fiber and micronutrients. I suggest eating different varieties of fruit. There are so many nutritional advantages to fruit, and most people do not eat enough of either fruits or vegetables.

My desire for something sweet used to come after dinner. If you desire something sweet as part of your meal, mix some fruit into your food, steamed veggies, or whatever. Get creative and have fun. Balsamic vinegar is sweet (sweet grape base), and I used to add it to many foods early on. A sudden increase in fruit intake can cause gas and bloating due to the fiber, so add gradually. The bloating and flatulence are temporary.

ALCOHOL (CONCURRENT WITH ELIMINATING SUGAR)

I can already hear the moans and groans. "Do I have to give up my glass of wine and my martinis?" The answer is yes, and for now, think of it as temporary. Alcohol is very similar to processed sugar when it comes to the effects on your body and brain. It's addictive, and your body has an inflammatory response. Drinking alcoholic beverages and eating processed sugar are both sources of brain fog and increase your risk of diabetes and other diseases. So yes, when you eliminate sugar from your diet, please do yourself a favor and eliminate alcoholic beverages, at least for the first four to six weeks.

Some studies[9] show a direct relationship between drinking (alcohol) and binging or disordered eating. The explanation is that alcohol's effect on insulin will actually increase hunger. Secondarily, if you're somebody who struggles with overeating, alcohol will also reduce your ability to control this behavior.

No, you don't have to swear off alcohol forever, but you'll see the benefits of eliminating it as routine when you've given it up for a month or two. You're likely to have a lower tolerance for alcohol with reducing sugar intake, so if you choose to have a drink once in a while, you'll feel the effects more quickly and with greater severity. Substitutions include any non-alcoholic, unsweetened beverage of your choice.

PROCESSED FOODS

Next, I started to learn about processed foods. As they figured out how to make zero-calorie soda in the '60s, the big food companies have gone into their labs, and they've figured out how to create the same junk food with substitutes for gluten, sugar, and dairy. Often these foods are highly processed with ingredients that didn't even originate as a food product but something concocted in a lab. Buyer beware! It has become a fad (yes, in some cases, fad diets) to eliminate gluten, sugar, or dairy without understanding why you should eliminate these foods.

I became obsessed with reading the labels on anything packaged. If there were anything I couldn't pronounce or appeared to be derived in a lab, I wouldn't buy it. When you see something that you wouldn't eat or buy by itself as a WF product on an ingredients label, it's likely to have been added to enhance the flavor, feed a food addiction, or increase the shelf life. It's certainly not added to improve your health. Some examples are MSG, maltodextrin and 'natural flavor, to name a few.

I then learned about processed oils. While fats are required in your diet to digest and process carbohydrates and proteins properly, I decided that I'd only eat high-quality olive oil or avocado oil. Most of the other oils that foods are fried in are of lesser quality, highly processed and can wreak havoc on your microbiome. Packaged or bottled salad dressings are often made with highly processed oils and aren't healthy.

I was never a fan of fried foods, but I was obsessed with eating popcorn when I went to the movies. And, of course, that meant a big bucket all to myself. It became a joke between my husband and me. If we discussed going to the movies, I always had to check my plans for the next day. I was certain to have a royal stomach ache. I learned that this was probably due to the oil they used to pop the popcorn and GMO corn.

Substitutions and adjustments that made my journey easier included extending my frozen yogurt shops to be gourmet popcorn bars. We popped the organic popcorn in-house using organic avocado oil and sprayed it lightly with olive oil so that the salt or any of the other 25 powdered organic flavors would stick. I now own my own popcorn machine at home, make a few buckets at a time, and often gift much of it to friends and family.

I also introduced nut milk frozen yogurt into the yogurt shops, and I was off and running. I was learning how to find healthier ways to eat the foods I loved. This was so exciting. Oh yes, my taste buds were dancing, my health and energy were improving, and, you guessed it, the scale was gradually tracking lower numbers.

ANIMAL PRODUCTS

As I mentioned earlier in the book, I now adhere to WFPB food choices, with no animal products. In the next chapter, I'll discuss why I chose to go that way and why I suggest you consider the same.

I've hesitated to discuss this until now because I don't want to say you can't eat animal products and still be healthy and maintain your healthy weight. However, this wasn't an option for me.

I'm not comfortable trusting myself to define moderation, so I pretty much adhere to WFPB to help me make decisions about what I eat.

 TIP:

The doctors and nutritionists who I respect who promote a plant-centric diet, including animal protein, suggest that the animal protein be no more than 10% of your total diet.

The topic of cholesterol has become a bit controversial, almost in a religious or political sense. People look for supporting arguments about cholesterol being problematic or not. The truth is you can find plenty of arguments on either side. Most recently, Simon Hill authored *The Proof is in the Plants*, citing many credible and unbiased studies that confirm that cholesterol is directly related to the high incidence of atherosclerosis or heart disease. Furthermore, as a result of his research, he believes that we should be considering a Low-Density Lipoproteins (LDL) of under 50, rather than the accepted 100 it is now, as a healthy level. This is where it's been shown to reduce our risk of heart disease.

In addition to cholesterol, processed meats and red meat have an inflammatory compound. Some who argue that cholesterol isn't so bad will admit that the inflammation in our heart and blood system is the real risk to large quantities of meat. Animal products in the quantity that make up the SAD absolutely increase the risk for diabetes, high blood pressure, high cholesterol, heart disease, stroke, depression, dementia, anxiety, autoimmune diseases and more.

I want to be completely transparent about my journey pursuing optimum health and weight. I did reach a point where I believed that would only come if I eliminated all animal products, and most of the research that I continue to review indicates the same, and yes, some would argue the opposing point of view with research to back it up.

Substitutions include tofu, though this isn't an option for me. I do not care for it. I do love mushrooms. I never knew about the many varieties of mushrooms. They have a consistency that's a great substitution for meat, and they absorb the flavor of whatever herbs and spices you use to prepare them. They're my number one go-to. Jackfruit is another very popular substitute for meat in many recipes. I've discovered many beans and legumes that add substance, protein, and fiber to any meal. I also make a lot of sauces with nuts and beans that are wonderful. Eggplant is another food I've loved but didn't eat often. Now it's another staple.

TIP:

Sometimes, you may eat out of habit. If you can identify appropriate substitutions for the foods you're giving up, you have the opportunity to create new healthier habits.

HYDRATION, HYDRATION, HYDRATION

I mentioned how important drinking water is when I discussed nutrition in Chapter IV. It's not only important for your body, but it's also helpful in your journey. Water makes you feel full, and therefore if you drink water with meals, you're less likely to miss the signals that you're satisfied.

If you take water with you at all times, you're helping your body digest and function more efficiently. If you think you're craving food, drinking water will help the cravings to disappear.

Finally, and this was *big* for me, when you're eating and you're so excited about what you're tasting and want more even though your body is telling you you've had enough, the water dilutes the taste on your tongue and helps you listen to your body.

NOT NECESSARILY ALWAYS AND FOREVER

Once you've gone a couple of months without many of the less healthy foods you previously had eaten, you'll probably find that you prefer the substitutes you've discovered. However, you may still be interested in a few of the less processed foods from your past. The difference is that the interest in those foods is no longer an addiction or a must-have. Now you can practice 'moderation,' and I mean true moderation. I would still recommend staying away from highly processed foods for good. You'll be rewarded with completely losing a taste for them if you do.

I still eat clean, dark chocolate occasionally, and I'll have a few drinks throughout the year. It never feels like an obsession. It's a choice because it's something that tastes good, and I'm satisfied with a small portion. If you want me to tell you that you can eat those Pringles you love once in a while, yes, you can. However, I believe you won't want to because they just won't taste good.

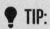 **TIP:**

This is the most important tip for your successful journey. Take the time to find healthy substitutes for the unhealthy, processed foods you've been eating.

IT'S SO SIMPLE, BUT IT'S NOT ALWAYS EASY

As discussed earlier in the book, your journey will help you accomplish two things. One is freedom from your previously toxic relationship with food. If you stay true to yourself for several months, you'll be amazed how the psychological and emotional aspect of eating that had you feeling imprisoned for so many years seems to be far less of an issue. The second is the improved physical and mental health that comes from eating healthy foods. Hippocrates' quote, "Let food be thy medicine," starts to become crystal clear.

Set yourself up for success. Make short-term commitments to yourself. I know it's hard to believe that this will be anything but another diet for some. You may be thinking that it'll be a trial, at best, of how long you can deprive yourself this time. If you're willing to do the 'cold turkey one food category at a time' approach to reduce your cravings, you'll start feeling better, and you'll start thinking about it differently.

Always, always have clean food options available that you love. This means planning. If you're traveling, keep in mind that airports do *not* have food you'll want to eat. Know how long you'll be away from home running errands, or know your plans for food on any given day at the office. If you do clean up your diet, you'll suffer the consequences when you find you need to eat unhealthy foods because you didn't plan ahead

TAKE THIS JOURNEY WITH A FRIEND

Let's face it, eating is now, and always will be, a social activity. There are many good ways to handle social situations and keep true to yourself. Is a night out eating the wrong foods worth a stomach ache and feeling bloated for a week or more afterward?

If you take this journey with a friend, you have someone to share the experiences of creating delicious, healthy recipes or exploring new restaurants. You have someone you can talk to when it's in the early weeks of giving up sugar, and you're still craving that chocolate cake because you've just dealt with a stressful situation at work.

When you're there for your friend, you'll find that nothing makes you feel better than when you can help another person. Supporting someone else's journey lends an extra boost of support for your own journey. Sometimes you'll hold up your friend, and sometimes they'll come to your rescue. That part of a relationship is more valuable than the chocolate cake you'd otherwise share with your friends. You owe it to yourself and each other. You can both relate to the stories that led you to this point in time.

BE YOUR OWN 'BFF'

Start practicing self-love if you really can't find someone interested in taking this journey with you. Rather than bullying yourself about this one area where you feel you've not attained the goals you set for yourself, dig deep and find the person inside that you'd be for a friend needing support. Now that you understand it wasn't your lack of willpower or discipline that had you fail, do you think you can find the 'best friend forever' we all should be for ourselves?

YOUR HOUSEMATE ISN'T INTERESTED IN YOUR JOURNEY

How do you handle things when the person you live with isn't on the same journey that you're on? I'd like to say, heck with them, but it's not that simple. I happened to be, and I still am, that person. For the years we raised our three sons, my husband has always done the grocery shopping and cooking. I never stopped appreciating that he did that, both because he loved to cook and because I was afraid of my lack of control around food. I had a love-hate (mostly hate) relationship with food for so many years.

When I decided to diet or starve myself, and I wasn't eating the food my husband prepared for all of us, he took it personally. So, you can imagine how freaked out he was when

I stopped eating bread, cheese, and pasta. Initially, he took it all in stride and started making chicken dishes every night. But then I eliminated animal products from my diet. He felt like I was rejecting *him*, not just the foods he was preparing. He believed he brought a nurturing value to our relationship, but part of this identity was now wounded.

He had no interest in changing the way he ate. He still doesn't. He eats animal products and processed foods. The further I got into my journey, the less it bothered me that he could sometimes be sarcastic about my choices. The better I felt and looked, the harder it was for me to understand how he could continue eating the way he did. But there was a lesson for both of us. We learned to support and respect each other and allowed the space to make our personal choices for ourselves.

Now I love to cook, and we make different versions of the same dinner every night. I'm having a blast. I love going to the grocery store, cooking and preparing my vegan meals. And he still has a lot of things to teach me in the kitchen too.

CREATE A SUPPORT SYSTEM

I know many recovering alcoholics who have been sober for many years still regularly attend meetings (12-step programs). The individual reasons are varied, but they all boil down to support and accountability. Programs such as these allow you to reflect on your behavior and your choices. You're also participating in these meetings with people with whom you have at least one thing in common, and that's your particular affliction or addiction.

If it's overeating you struggle with, there is a 12-step program for that. If you're on this journey, it'd be wonderful for the other attendants if you were to share your successes.

If you don't think you fit into an existing support group, you can set one up. I guarantee you know many other people who would like to have a better relationship with food. If they do not realize they have food issues and struggle with obesity, heart disease, cancer, or just about any other ailment, they'd be the perfect person to include.

We've now all figured out that technology allows us to connect with people regardless of their geographic location. Use social media to network with people that want to take this journey with you. There are so many online meetings available right now, so there's no excuse not to join. Just find or create your support group.

You're embarking on a major life event. Make no mistake. This is a lifestyle change. This is different from other support groups for substance abuse because once you've built a healthy relationship with food, you'll probably not go back to your old way of eating. If you proceed on this journey with a friend or create a support group, it'll probably end up being more of a social gathering where you can discuss which organized run you're signing up for or all the wonderful recipes you're creating.

You won't need to attend meetings to stay on track for months and years to come. The challenge is only in the beginning months when you're adjusting to this new lifestyle, gradually altering one food group at a time and adopting a new way to eat. Then you'll observe how many other things in your life change for the better.

ALWAYS HAVE CLEAN FOOD OPTIONS AVAILABLE

When I proceeded on my journey to healthy eating, I had to change how I shopped for food. I had to plan meals ahead of time, and I had to explore new recipes. I had not been responsible for any of these things for years. I agreed to a four-to-six-week cold turkey period with each change I decided to make. It didn't require me going through the refrigerator or pantry and throwing away everything that may have tempted me, but if you need to do this, do it. If you live with someone else whose less healthy foods will remain in the house, ask them if it's okay to keep these items tucked away so they won't be visible every time you open the pantry.

It may be true that breakfast is the most important meal of the day. I should note that eating breakfast every day was new for me. In the past, if I ate breakfast, it somehow triggered me to be hungrier throughout the day. Could it have been those darn empty calories in most breakfast foods that spike your insulin?

It was a challenge for me to find interesting foods for breakfast. I'd started eating almond butter on GF, wholegrain crackers every morning for breakfast. I also started having to travel quite a bit. That creates a challenge for food throughout the day for a GF WFPB eater. Carrying around almond butter on crackers doesn't work well. I discovered a gap in the market for super clean, GF, vegan packaged foods.

READ THE INGREDIENTS

Spoiler alert. This is where I shamelessly plug my new business, Read The Ingredients, launched with Michael, my business partner and oldest son.

I set out to bake a WFPB, unsweetened, GF, mini loaf that would be hearty enough to be a full breakfast or lunch meal and would travel well. I also created another product equally portable, equally healthy, and great for snacking throughout the day. Today those products are widely available online and will be available in retail stores in 2022. The brand name is Read The Ingredients (rtifoods.com). It was important that if I were going to be true to myself and commit to my relationship with food, I had to have foods that were packaged (but not processed) for convenience and that I would want to eat, at the ready, at all times.

In 2018, Michael and I were thinking about selling our frozen yogurt business. We shared our products with others who had a commitment to healthy eating and received very enthusiastic feedback. We realized there was a market for these products. There is nothing as clean, tasty, conveniently packaged and portable on the market as our products. Our company, Read The Ingredients, was born. It's gratifying to know that our products promote and help people build a healthier lifestyle.

We intended to convey two important messages to people who seriously consider their relationship with food. Firstly, do not put yourself in a situation where you'll get hungry and need to grab something you shouldn't and don't want to eat. *Always* have clean options available. If you get stuck and find yourself eating some crappy, processed food, you may risk a setback. To this day, if I'm going out, running errands and think I may get hungry, I grab nuts, fruit, or Read The Ingredients products to take along with me.

The second message is, if you're eating packaged food, read the ingredients! Know what you're putting in your body and make your choices accordingly.

WHAT'S NEXT

It should be starting to make sense how different this is than the dieting efforts from years past. Rather than spending energy and counting the days until you can stop depriving yourself, you spend the early, more challenging weeks exploring foods that you can eat as healthy substitutes. It's a whole new world to explore. This gives your microbiome, hormones, and taste buds time to reset. You'll start getting very excited about how much better you feel. You'll forget that you ever thought you'd miss those sandwich cookies that you've been eating for so many years.

While giving you my step-by-step journey that transformed my toxic relationship with food into a wonderful one, I admit that I tread lightly on the topic of giving up animal products completely. I admit that people I know say they must include some animal protein to feel healthy. Again, I don't have a professional background to insist otherwise. I only have my own experience and the research I've done.

Please keep in mind the importance of setting up your environment and your social network to be supported. This is particularly important in the early weeks and months of your journey. With that said, I've dedicated Chapter VI to my commitment to a vegan lifestyle and 100% plant-based eating. Please understand I'm not preaching. I'm not nagging. I'm sharing my personal beliefs, and I'm very clear that I spent 57 years of my life with little awareness of what moved the needle for me.

Please proceed with curiosity and with no guilt or shame. I'm just sharing my relatively recently developed philosophy.

"Whatever makes you uncomfortable is your biggest opportunity for growth."

—Bryant H. McGill

CHAPTER V EXERCISE:

Refer to the lists that you created in Chapter IV exercise. See if there is a common theme among the foods that do not make you feel well, that you constantly crave, or feel you have an addiction.

1. What food group are you going to eliminate first? Starting when?

    a. What substitutes do you have for that food?

    b. List what you notice four to six weeks after you've eliminated those foods.

2. What food group are you going to eliminate second?

    a. Starting when?

    b. What substitutes do you have for that food?

    c. List what you notice four to six weeks after you've eliminated those foods.

3. Repeat the above each time you're ready to eliminate another food group. I suggest you eliminate one at a time, giving each four to eight weeks before moving onto the next one.

CHAPTER VI

LET'S TALK ABOUT THE ANIMALS

"The love for all living creatures is the most noble attribute of man."

—Charles Darwin

INTRODUCTION

Before going any further, I must warn you. If you're hell-bent on not giving up animal products, I get it. You can choose to skip this chapter if you feel that strongly. Or, if you think you can read it just to get a sense of another person's experience (mine) as they ventured fully into the vegan world, then approach this chapter with that mindset.

If you do decide to skip this chapter, and you're still intrigued enough by the information that I've shared to this point, then I hope that you'll proceed on your journey. Maybe one day, when you feel less overwhelmed about the prospect of reducing your consumption or giving up animal products completely, you'll return to read this chapter then. My point is, do *not* throw out the baby with the bathwater. Yes, you can improve your relationship with food without 100% giving up animal products.

MEET PEOPLE WHERE THEY ARE

I have a confession. I've purposely presented this book about my journey without overly emphasizing that I now eat only plant-based foods. I live a vegan lifestyle.

The following story reminds me how divisive the topic of veganism can be. About 15 years ago, when I moved to a more rural area of California, I needed a new doctor. Not being fond of doctors in general, I asked around for referrals. I was told that this one doctor leaned more towards homeopathy in both treatments and philosophy. That was a plus because I was already aware and resented that most doctors resorted to 'Big Pharma' drugs. Knowing that I'm super sensitive to any chemicals I put in my body, I've never been a fan of drugs.

I walked into this doctor's office and gave her my history, including that I often felt tired, rundown, bloated and constipated. I was still very much of the mindset that I'd been eating healthy except for my diet soda addiction. Within the first five minutes in her office, she recommended eliminating all animal products from my diet. She gave me very little explanation as to why she was suggesting that. It was like a blow to the head. I don't remember anything else she said, or even if she did say anything else. My brain went straight to the image of my husband's face when I walked through the door and told him the doctor prescribed veganism. I knew he'd be so upset if I were even to consider it. I hung on to that thought all the way home. I went into my house, told him, and received my expected reaction. I didn't give it another thought for about six years.

The lesson is to meet people where they are. Without giving me any other information about *why* I should become vegan, she didn't have a chance of convincing me. Likewise, I don't want to come at you with something that seems so radical that you won't even consider it.

While I do believe that this journey can't be complete if animal products are still a big part of your diet, I know that any steps in that general direction will be positive. As I said in Chapter V, there are well-documented examples of people who seem to accomplish what my journey afforded me by including no more than 10% of their total diet being animal protein.

With more than 10% animal products in your nutritional lifestyle, it would be challenging to accomplish all your goals. It'll be difficult to have an outstanding relationship with food that will lead you down the path of a very healthy, energized, vital life for as long as you live.

I appreciate that you've allowed me to share an aspect of my journey that I believe made all the difference in achieving a rich, healthy and joyful relationship with food. I believe that plant protein is better for us because it does not come with any of the negative effects of animal protein, such as high cholesterol, inflammation and heart disease.

It's debated that animal protein sources offer more complete proteins, which is true in many cases. However, it's absolutely possible and quite simple to get complete protein by combining plants.

There's one other ironic example in my life that proves many people don't always connect the dots until they're ready. In 1995 my stepmother, Sandy, died of Mad Cow Disease. When the disease presents in humans, it's called Creutzfeldt-Jakob Disease (CJD). This is a rare disease, so it became a major news event when it was discovered in the UK in the 80s & 90s.

Interestingly, except for UK exported beef, there was little reduction in beef consumption. But if you witnessed the course this terminal disease takes, as I did, it's unbelievable to me that all of us, her friends and family, did not immediately eliminate meat from our diets.

Yes, this discussion can only be heard when you're ready for it. In 1995 when my stepmother, Sandy, died, I wasn't ready to reflect on my own nutritional lifestyle. However, 15 years later, I was ready to do and try anything to restore my health, energy, and the confidence that I'd have a great quality of life, however long I lived.

> Meet people where they are. Something made you pick up this book. You told yourself it was your time to take back control and quality of your life. Respect that everyone starts that journey when they're ready.

DEFINING DIFFERENT FOOD PREFERENCES

Let me arm you with an understanding of the different eating methods. This will enable you to engage in the conversation. This is different than specific trends and diets that you may hear about that I discussed in Chapter III (i.e., Keto and Paleo):

- Omnivores eat animals and plants.
- Vegetarians do not eat animal products where the animal must be killed, such as meat, but they may

eat dairy, eggs, and other animal products where the animal does not die to provide.

- Flexitarians lean toward a vegetarian diet but eat meat occasionally.

- Pescatarians eat fish but no other meat. Eggs and dairy are also acceptable for some.

- Vegans consume no animal products in the foods they eat, the clothes they wear (no leather), the sundries they buy (no animal testing), and may or may not subscribe to 'clean eating.' Thus the term 'junk food vegans.'

- WFPB foods have no animal products and no processed foods.

- Whole30 is initially presented as a food plan (experiment) to eat only whole foods for 30 days to readjust your system. It emphasizes whole foods without the exclusion of animal products. Also, the Whole30 plan excludes all sugars, grains and legumes, including pseudo-cereal products such as quinoa, amaranth and others.

THE IMPORTANCE OF CLEAN EATING

To reiterate, the difference between WFPB and Whole30 choices and any other choices listed above is that those who adopt WFPB or Whole30 lifestyles will avoid processed foods. It's important to eliminate preservatives and additives of any kind. That's the top priority.

With the absence of the right nutrients in processed foods, you're likely to eat a lot more calories and become addicted to unhealthy choices. Likewise, animal products are calorically dense with saturated fats. These are the reasons for you to consider transitioning to a WFPB lifestyle.

My experience (and it is well documented[10] that it's the experience of many others) is that this is the easiest way to maintain a healthy weight. You may eat a lot more food, but you'll consume fewer calories and no empty calories. If you learn to select and prepare foods to keep your choices interesting, you'll feel satiated, and your cravings for unhealthy and processed foods will disappear. You'll look forward to the flavorful new foods and recipes you've discovered.

HEART HEALTH

The doctors I believe in and the studies I've reviewed present evidence that the amount of saturated fat consumed with animal products is why we have such a high incidence of heart disease and strokes. Published studies[11] indicate that heart disease can be prevented and even reversed by eliminating animal products and processed foods. Often these doctors prescribe a change in diet for their patients rather than the more traditional drugs for high cholesterol and high blood pressure with great success.

YOUR IMMUNE SYSTEM

Processed foods are the biggest disruptors of your microbiome. A healthy immune system needs fiber. When food is processed, there is no fiber left. The people with the weakest immune systems are those whose diets are fiber deficient. Animal products do not offer any fiber. With WFPB foods, the densest plant protein is found in beans, lentils, and other legumes. These foods also have a great deal of fiber.

ANIMALS SAVED MY LIFE (RETURNING THE FAVOR)

Nowadays, I tell others I came to this lifestyle for my health, but I stayed for the animals and my grandchildren. Let me explain. I've always loved animals. When I grew up in my less than happy home, my parents brought home our first dog, Scarlett, a beautiful Irish Setter, when I was 13 years old. By then, I'd probably brought home at least half a dozen strays, only to have Sandy, my stepmother, toss them out of the house.

I swear Scarlett was my salvation. She'd sleep on my bed every night. I'd wake up in the morning to her beautiful brown eyes looking at me lovingly and letting me know she was ready to start the day. I was the one person in our house who would take her out for walks and feed her. Whenever I was home, she was my constant companion. I had a connection with her and have had with every one of my animals since. I trusted them. After all, animals are honest and transparent about how they feel. They also sense our energy and how we feel. I don't know about you, but I can't say this is so with most people I grew up around. My pets have been an important part of my life and our family ever since.

Despite this love for animals, it never dawned on me what life was like for commercially raised animals. As I embarked on my journey and moved strongly towards veganism, I became interested in the many documentaries produced that reveal the horrendous conditions and suffering on these farms and ranches. I know that I can never go back to any other way of eating.

The truth is that I feel like animals gave me a chance at life, including all the strays I picked up as a child, and my first real forever pet, Scarlett. They continue to be such an integral part of my day. With the four horses, four dogs, and three cats that make up my current four-legged family members, my life and attitude about animals have been transformed forever.

For years, all the dogs and cats we've had have been rescues that needed a home. For me, it's more than a cliché to ask the question, who is rescuing who. This is where I go for calmness and connection. My horses are my retreat when I'm having a bad day, or every chance I have to make it an even better day. The least I can do is my part in giving them their life back. I feel strongly that we've no need and no right to raise animals, often in unnatural and deplorable conditions, just to slaughter them for food we don't need to eat.

THE PLANET

Wherever you live, take note of the climate change we're all experiencing. Until recently, most people have had the attitude "the sun will come up tomorrow," and all will be fine. That's no longer the case. It's been proven that the methane gas produced by the agriculture industry is consistently one of the top 3 offenders to climate change and global warming[12].

All around our planet, there are problems due to the changing climate. I think I always subconsciously figured "nothing disastrous will happen in my lifetime." That may still be the case. But once I became a grandparent and realized even if my generation gets through this unscathed, my children's and grandchildren's generations almost certainly won't.

What kind of planet are we leaving for future generations? If shrinking the impact on the planet is possible by reducing the demand for animal products, that's reason enough for me to commit to the lifestyle that gave me my life back.

DOING GOOD

As I've mentioned previously, my life has been transformed by my journey, and writing this book is one of the ways I'm paying it forward. In my mind, nothing feels better than selflessly and selfishly giving back to others. I'm proud to share my strong beliefs about a vegan lifestyle and speak out for the animals who can't speak out for themselves. We'd live in a wonderful world if everybody did one small selfless act each day. It may just help you not have to ever think about your weight again.

WHAT'S NEXT

In the next chapter, I'll proudly and with humility share with you how my life changed drastically within the first year of my journey and how it just keeps getting better. Know that I wish this for you and much more.

"I said somebody should do something about that, and then I realized I am somebody."

—Unknown

CHAPTER VI EXERCISE:

Decide if you want to entertain any of the following documentaries to understand fully the reasons why you should consider removing animal products from your menu:

- The Game Changers
- Forks Over Knives
- Cowspiracy
- What the Health
- Seaspiracy
- Vegucated
- Rotten
- The Milk System

CHAPTER VII

WHAT DOES IT FEEL LIKE TO HAVE A HEALTHY RELATIONSHIP WITH FOOD?

"Every success story is a tale of constant adaption, revision and change."

—Richard Branson

INTRODUCTION

Congratulations! You've made it this far into the book. Now for the rewards.

Within a couple of months, the hard part of the journey exists in the rearview mirror. In retrospect, I had a few days that I just had to be strong and say no, but for all the rewards and the fact that I'm not interested in eating anything other than WFPB choices, this journey has been worthwhile and a huge success.

Overall, the biggest reward is getting your life back! Now that you're not spending time dwelling on all things food, weight and appearance (i.e., a toxic relationship with food), we've made room to deal with more important projects in life. Certainly, we've made room to experience more joy.

CRAVINGS (ADDICTIONS) ARE GONE

I no longer have any interest in the unhealthy foods I used to eat. Cravings for sweets and salty foods are a thing of the past. You may have read that last sentence and thought, "Who is she kidding?" Okay, that's fair, so I want to give you an example.

The old me was obsessed with chocolate, specifically milk chocolate. I'd have a conversation about it before, during, and after eating it. When I'd decide to eat chocolate, which in my opinion back then wasn't often enough, I'd eat as much as I could get my hands on. I'd tell myself, "I don't do this often, so go ahead, indulge!" The conversation during eating was, "This tastes so good, but I know I'm going to pay the price when I try to get out of bed tomorrow." Now I wonder, with all this noise in my head, did I even taste the chocolate, or was it something I thought I was tasting? Then for days afterward, constipated and bloated, I'd promise myself I'd never do this again. Of course, I did eat chocolate again, and then, I'd beat myself up for being a liar, going back on a promise, and having no willpower.

Today, I truly love dark chocolate. I eat it maybe once or twice a month. It does not call to me. Rather it's a conscious choice to open the refrigerator, grab a small amount and enjoy the treat. Interestingly, I don't think of it as a treat. It's just the delicious food that I'll eat at that moment. While I'm slowly chewing and enjoying, it's nothing but pleasurable.

Everything is different now. My husband's ice cream doesn't call to me from the freezer anymore. The chips he bought weeks ago are sitting in my pantry unopened, and strangely I have no interest in them. I look at meat with a bit of distaste,

TIP:

Have you heard of the 'ick factor' (made famous in an episode of the TV show Sex in the City)? It's when suddenly, everything about your partner bothers you or makes you cringe about the way they eat, the way they brush their teeth, etc. There will likely become a point when your relationship to the unhealthy foods you were eating will feel like that. Your appetite for those foods will go away.

but I do not let it affect me. For example, I can enjoy a meal with my husband, regardless of what he's eating.

I'M NO LONGER A MOODY B**CH

While I firmly believe that my first two marriages were mistakes, I often wonder what kind of relationships I would have had if I'd been on this journey when I was considerably younger. Even I can acknowledge I was pretty dang moody!

Earlier, I shared about good days and bad days being tied to my weight, how my clothes fit, feeling bloated or eating too much. The moodiness was quite apparent on my bad days. I had a lot less patience with people around me. I was easily frustrated. I'd become annoyed at the simplest things. Yes, it's a fact that the foods you eat can affect your moods and can even cause serious bouts of depression. I'm not kidding. This is different if you adopt a WFPB approach to food. If you don't believe me, ask my husband!

FEELING SAFE

For many years, I'd wake up wondering if it would be a good day. A good or bad day was determined by how hungry I felt and what foods I chose to eat or which size suit I pulled out of my closet to wear to work. It was a good day when I knew I had the stuff to make a salad in the refrigerator for when I got home, so I didn't have to go to the grocery store. Going to the grocery store never happened on a good day, and if it did, it often turned a good day into a bad day. Now, I finally feel safe in my body.

Food is still a big part of any day, but it's been years since my days are turned bad based on the food I've eaten that day. I feel safe going to the grocery store, going to friends' houses for dinner, or going to a restaurant. Our large family Thanksgiving dinners are now safe, as it's no longer a given that I'll go to bed in pain because of the four desserts I would've eaten in the past.

SOCIAL EVENTS

As an introvert, social gatherings aren't my favorite thing to do. In the past attending a party would wreak havoc on my mental state. This was not because I was uncomfortable around people. I'm not. But social situations meant food and drink. I was always monitoring my response to the food.

To quiet my thoughts, I'd choose to drink. My brain would spin. Do I want to suffer a hangover (that doesn't take much for me)? Do I want to lose control of what I'm going to eat out of boredom, trying to fit in, or anxiety? This was my brain at a party.

Now, food is a non-issue. I'm still an introvert but not shy (this means I get energized mostly with things I do alone or with one other person). If I choose to attend a social gathering, there is no chance I'll have a food issue. I no longer crave the foods that I don't eat. If I believe the social gathering won't have any suitable foods, I make sure I fill up beforehand, so I don't go hungry. While it's still not my favorite thing to do, if I attend a social gathering, it won't be a night that I'll regret, at least not in the way I used to.

ENERGIZED

I'm in my mid-60s, and I have more energy and do more in a day now than I did in my 40s. My husband and I spend 45 minutes in our gym first thing every morning. I'm building and running my own business with my son and business partner, Michael. I play two to three hours of aggressive pickleball several times a week, and I spend hours every week with my horses. When I have time, I ski in the winter and ride my bike in the summer. Twenty years ago, I would've been exhausted just thinking about doing this many things in a day, week or month.

I'm committed to being the 'cool' grandmother who gets a chance to ski with her grandchildren. I've always been very active. But 20 years ago I didn't have the energy I do now, and of course, I weighed 20 to 30 pounds more, and I found it challenging to get a good night's sleep. My WFPB lifestyle was the key for me, and I believe it is for most people.

CONFIDENCE

I believe I'm not alone having uttered, "If I were thin, life would be so much better, and I really believe I could have it all." If you have your health, you *could* have it all. That potential is realized when you feel confident. Honestly, I haven't lacked confidence (sometimes bordering on arrogance) for many years. However, there was always that nagging feeling of, "If I'm so confident that I can do anything, why can't I lose weight and look the way I want to look?"

I now know it wasn't about the weight. It was about how I felt. When you lack the energy to live the life you want, you start doubting your abilities.

BETTER RELATIONSHIPS WITH FAMILY AND FRIENDS

I don't think many people can say that they haven't been guilty of snapping at their children, spouse or coworkers when they're having a bad day. This happens a lot because they're in a bad mood, and sometimes they can't even identify why.

Now that I'm a less moody and frankly much happier person than before, I enjoy spending time with friends and family. It seems like the conversation is lighter, and being with others is a lot more fun. So, while I was consciously changing my relationship with food, I was vastly improving my relationships with those around me.

A NEW WAY OF THINKING

No gluten, no animal products, and no processed food. No guilt, no second-guessing, no going to sleep in pain, or waking up bloated and in worse pain. Now breakfast gives me the energy and focus I need to take on the day. It no longer means, "Oh, screw it. There goes my day. I may as well eat whatever I want and start over tomorrow."

I can identify when I'm genuinely hungry and when I'm eating for some other reason. On most days, I can honor my body when it tells me it's satisfied. When I choose to eat for reasons other than hunger, which I still do occasionally, there are no repercussions or consequences because what I eat is good for me.

I know you may be reading this with disbelief, and I'm sure I'd have had the same reaction ten years ago. But I promise you. I've never had a moment of missing a single food that I used to eat. Eating and just living are so much more fun.

> My journey offered me freedom from a toxic relationship with food, and I got my life back!

THE JOURNEY ISN'T OVER

When you finally feel confident that you understand how your food choices impact your emotions, you may just want to keep feeling better. As mentioned earlier, I'm constantly fine-tuning my balance of macronutrients and micronutrients.

The beauty of taking care of yourself is that you start to identify when things may become a bit off. If you feel like you're out of balance, you may want to have your doctor run a bloodwork panel for you, so you can see if you need any adjustments in your micronutrients or supplements. You may even decide to try a 24-hour fast or cleanse. Many people read about these things, and without evaluating their overall diet, they think this will solve the problem. It won't. But if you're eating clean, WFPB foods, this could be the icing on the cake.

As in life and all of your relationships, it's the journey that continues, and if you're mindful about how you proceed, you'll continue to move in a positive direction. We all have the same endpoint, so we may as well enjoy the ride for as long as we can.

YOU CAN HAVE IT ALL

As I said in the Introduction, my journey has taken me to a better life than I could've ever dreamed. I'm a fit grandmother of six, and I have a dream relationship with my adult children. My firstborn is my business partner and one of the best business partners I've ever had. I've been married to my husband for well over three decades, and I feel he's the one I'm thrilled to grow old with, despite that we're not on the same food journey.

But here's the best part. When most people are winding down in their 60s, I feel like I still have so much I want to do. I'm passionate about Read The Ingredients and the idea that we could support anyone on a similar food and lifestyle journey.

Mostly I feel that by removing the stress about food, my health and my weight, I have made room in my life for more of a spiritual element and a strong desire to be of service to others. I'm not sure how much room I had for that in the past when so much energy was spent just trying to stay healthy, find energy, and struggle with my previously toxic relationship with food. I've achieved the freedom I was seeking.

WHAT'S NEXT

Please keep reading. The next few sections of this book offer the following:

- The Tips and Tricks section explains what has worked to help me transition smoothly and painlessly into my WFPB lifestyle.
- The Endnotes section details the studies and research I've quoted throughout the book (I recommend you

read these to further your understanding of the topics covered in this book).

- The Resources section, so you continue feeling supported by professionals who share valuable information in books, social media, and blogs.
- The Keep in Touch section, where I'll give you my email address, and I look forward to hearing from you!

"Change is hard at first, messy in the middle and gorgeous at the end."

—Robin Sharma

CHAPTER VII EXERCISE:

1. Go back to your exercise in Chapter I to revisit your original goals and what motivated you to take this journey.

2. Every 30 to 45 days on your journey, note your progress! List what you feel good about your journey.

3. If you don't feel you're making your expected progress, list the reasons why not. If you feel it'd be helpful, revisit other exercises to get back on track.

4. If you want to reach out to me, please do. I offer my email address in the Keep in Touch section at the back of this book.

TIPS AND TRICKS

"When you recover or discover something that nourishes your soul and brings joy, care enough about yourself to make room for it in your life."

—Jean Shinoda Bolen

I've shared most of these tips throughout the book. I want to reiterate them here so, while you're on your journey, you can reference these to remind you of some of the tips that worked for me. Enjoy, and come up with more of your own that you share with me and others.

EARLY IN THE JOURNEY

Once you've committed to getting healthy and building a new, exciting relationship with food, you want to set yourself up for success. These are the tips that are critical during those early months:

- Remove the junk food from your house.

- Bring lots of clean, healthy snacks into your pantry, refrigerator, car, office, and where ever you spend extended periods.

- Always take water with you. Drink regularly. You should urinate every few hours, and it should be a very, very pale yellow. Anything darker, and you're not hydrated.

- Do not weigh yourself more frequently than once per week, or less frequently if you can stand it.

- Always have access to healthy whole foods. This would include GF food if you've given up gluten. Make a healthy trail mix with nuts and raisins. Grab an apple or banana on the way out the door.

- If you're craving food that you're removing from your diet, ask yourself why. Decide if you really are hungry, and then decide if you're going to eat. If so, decide what healthy food you'll eat.

- Do not determine how you look or feel based on Instagram pictures you see while scrolling. In fact, quit scrolling! In other words, how you look and feel shouldn't be based on a comparison to others.

- If you eliminate animal protein, and I hope you do, find substitutes that add texture and good nutrition to your plate. Mushrooms are my go-to food. I've discovered varieties of mushrooms I'd never eaten before.

- If you're afraid to commit to eliminating animal products, try committing to one meal a day that will be fully WFPB. Then take it further by picking two days next week to eliminate all animal products. Work yourself up slowly to a nearly or fully WFPB lifestyle. Once you've found that you can explore interesting meals and discover new plant-based foods that you're excited about, it'll be easier to let it all go.

- If sugar is particularly rough for you, eat fruit at whatever time of day you're triggered with a sugar urge. Eat as much fruit as you want in the beginning. Just beware. If your body isn't accustomed to having that much fiber, there will be repercussions with some gas and bloating. But you should feel full pretty quickly, and within a couple of weeks, those cravings for 'sweets' will subside.

- Always keep a list of 'lifelines' handy. You can phone a friend, take the dog for a walk, take up a new hobby, write a letter to your younger self, or whatever works for you.

AS YOU'RE ADJUSTING

- Introduce yourself to non-dairy milks, including nut, oat or soy. Check the ingredients if you are purchasing these in the store. Many of them are highly processed. So long as they're not, these milks are good for your coffee and great for making plant-based sauces. If you reach out to me, I can recommend an alternative, non-dairy milk appliance with which you can add water and make your own. Not only can you make all kinds of non-dairy milk much cleaner than what is sold in the stores, but you're also left with the pulp. I use this to make hummus, vegan mayonnaise, salad dressing, and pesto sauce for my GF pasta.

- I've never liked sautéing or frying food. I use the microwave quite a bit. I found I can cook mushrooms and lots of other vegetables with onions, garlic, herbs, and spices quickly in the microwave. There is a lot of information about the pros and cons of microwave cooking. One of the pros is that the faster you cook vegetables, the fewer nutrients are lost. I maintain the flavor, control how 'cooked' it comes out, and do not need to add any fat. I haven't yet tried one, but I think I'll eventually buy an air fryer.

- Redefine pizza. I used to love pizza. The cheesier, the better. I now make a 'killer' GF pizza crust that takes no time at all. I top my pizza with lots of vegetables and, of course, mushrooms. Tomato slices are my preference over pizza sauce. Sometimes I use lentils or beans mashed as a 'sauce' to hold the veggies. I've also used hummus under the veggies as a sauce substitute.

- As I mentioned in Chapter VII, my journey was ongoing while I reached my destination. Now that I have a very healthy relationship with food, I'm constantly fine-tuning what I eat. There are times when I feel my energy isn't what it should be. I look at things like my protein to carbs to fats ratios. I monitor my sleep quality and quantity. I constantly explore new plant-based foods and recipes. The difference now is that I continue down the path with excitement and enthusiasm. I know I'm expanding on the joy I'm experiencing in my relationship with food, others, and myself.

"Our bodies are our garden to which our wills are gardeners."

—William Shakespeare

ENDNOTES

1. https://www.ucsusa.org/resources/how-coca-cola-disguised-its-influence-science-about-sugar-and-health

   Also, inside *Hooked: How Processed Food Became Addictive* by Michael Moss (see Resources section)

2. https://www.medicalnewstoday.com/articles/cholesterol-research-does-industry-funding-skew-results

   https://www.pcrm.org/news/news-releases/new-review-study-shows-egg-industry-funded-research-downplays-danger-cholesterol

3. https://www.pcrm.org/good-nutrition/nutrition-information/health-concerns-with-eggs.

4. https://www.theatlantic.com/politics/archive/2016/05/low-tar-cigarettes/481116/

   Also, inside *Hooked: How Processed Food Became Addictive* by Michael Moss (see Resources section)

5. https://theplantfedgut.com/

   Also, inside *Fiber Fueled* by Dr. Will Bulsiewicz (see Resources section)

6. https://www.everydayhealth.com/diet-nutrition/metabolism-may-not-decline-with-age-as-previously-thought/

https://www.science.org/doi/10.1126/science.abe5017

7. *Inside The Unhealthy Truth: One Mother's Shocking Investigation into the Dangers of America's Food Supply – And What Every Family Can Do to Protect Itself* by Robyn O'Brien (see Resources section)

8. https://switch4good.org/

Also, Switch 4 Good podcast (see Resources section)

9. https://pubmed.ncbi.nlm.nih.gov/21208332/

https://www.eatingdisorderhope.com/information/binge-eating-disorder/binge-drinking-and-binge-eating-disorder-what-are-the-connections

10. https://www.forksoverknives.com/

11. *Food for Life and Your Body in Balance* by Dr. Neal Barnard

How to Not Die and *How to Not Diet* by Dr. Michael Greger

Program for Reversing Heart Disease and Undo It by Dr. Dean Ornish

Whole: Rethinking the Science of Nutrition by T. Colin Campbell

The Proof is in the Plants by Simon Hill

(see Resources section)

12. https://www.epa.gov/ghgemissions/global-greenhouse-gas-emissions-data

RESOURCES

As previously mentioned, I geek out on all things health-related and nutrition-related. Below you'll find some of the best sources I learned from and those that motivated me on my journey.

Please share with me if you find others that motivate you.

The benefits of a WFPB lifestyle:

- ○ Dr. Neal Barnard
  - *Food for Life*
  - *Your Body in Balance*

- ○ Dr. Michael Greger
  - *How to Not Die*
  - *How to Not Diet*

- ○ Dr. Dean Ornish
  - *Program for Reversing Heart Disease*
  - *Undo It*

- ○ T. Colin Campbell, Ph.D. Biochemist
  - *Whole: Rethinking the Science of Nutrition*

- ○ Simon Hill, Physiotherapist & Nutritionist
  - *The Proof is in the Plants*

The one diet book author I can suggest if you're not interested in becoming completely plant-based:

o Dr. Mark Hyman
  • *The Pegan Diet: 21 Practical Principles for Reclaiming Your Health in a Nutritionally Confusing World*

The importance of fiber:

o Dr. Will Bulsiewicz
  • *Fiber Fueled*

If you want to read more about food addiction:

o Michael Moss (investigative journalist)
  • *Hooked: How Processed Food Became Addictive*

o Dr. Anne Lembke (about general addiction)
  • *Dopamine Nation: Finding Balance in the Age of Indulgence*

Highly rated cookbooks focused on WFPB recipes:

o *Thug Kitchen: Eat Like You Give a F**k*
o *Thug Kitchen 101: Fast as F*ck*

I always recommend you purchase highly rated cookbooks because, even if you aren't committed to going 100% plant-based, these books will help you reduce the amount of animal protein you include in your meals.

My sons gave me the two Thug Kitchen books, and I can vouch that the recipes are easy, and you'll be introduced to many basics to create delicious WFPB meals. The language is X-rated. Buyer beware.

Podcasts:

I confess, I learned a lot from listening to the guests on these different podcasts, with Rich Roll's being number one for me. If you want to tune into podcasts that cover topics related to health and healthy eating:

○ Rich Roll Podcast by Rich Roll

(discussions with guests who are all about health and lifestyle)

○ The Exam Room by Chuck Carroll

(examines vegan nutrition and medical news)

○ Switch 4 Good by Dotsie Bausch and Alexandra Paul

(discussions regarding living a full, healthy, and joyous life through the foods we eat and our relationship to those foods)

TEDx Talks:

• Robyn O'Brien – two TEDx talks reveal why and how the food companies are feeding us toxic food (a must-listen). Robyn has also been interviewed on many podcasts. Her work is heroic, in my opinion.

• Robyn is also the author of The Unhealthy Truth: One Mother's Shocking Investigation into the Dangers of America's Food Supply – And What Every Family Can Do to Protect Itself.

Blogs and Websites (free subscriptions to informative email newsletters):

• ForksOverKnives.com - There is so much available from this site. They publish recipes that give me ideas of the basics, and then I can throw my version of many foods together. These recipes are basic enough that I feel "they teach me to fish rather than giving me the fish." Yes, there is some irony in the relevance of that cliché!

- FoodRevolution.org - John Robbins and son, Ocean Robbins' organization. If you don't know John Robbins' story, it's fascinating. He had the opportunity to be the heir to the Baskin-Robbins fortune. How's that for irony? You can search for the podcasts that have hosted and interviewed him, or you can read his book.

I've found some specific products and kitchen tools that have become invaluable to me and make WFPB food preparation easier. I've also discovered some foods that aren't readily found in many grocery stores. So I purchase these online and keep them in my pantry. I'd love to share these ideas with anyone who asks. If this is interesting to you, go to the Keep in Touch section at the end of this book and reach out to me.

KEEP IN TOUCH

I know your heart is in this, or you wouldn't have read this far in the book. You dare to take responsibility for your health. You're embarking on your own journey to learn how changing your relationship with food can be more effective in boosting your long-term vitality and quality of life than the medicine that doctors will offer.

As I said before, this is quite simple, but it's not easy. My health was such a motivator for me that there was no turning back. Because it made such a remarkable difference in my life, I'm compelled to share it with anyone interested in gaining freedom from a toxic relationship with food and starting their journey to an outstanding relationship.

I'd be honored and inspired to hear from anyone committed to experiencing their own transformation. If you're looking for someone to celebrate with you, understand your struggles, or share more secrets to success, please reach out to me at:

Freedom@RTIfoods.com

If you're interested in following our brand, Read The Ingredients, and the information-packed blogs on our website, go to:

RTIfoods.com

We share weekly blogs and newsletters on all things related to clean eating and living a healthy lifestyle.

I want to hear about your journey. I especially want to hear if you found things that worked for you, *really* worked to give you your life back.

I want to offer support. If you're looking to go deeper into the information in this book, I may be able to suggest other resources.

If you take exception with anything I've said in this book, I look forward to a healthy dialogue.

If you just want to brag or share about how you struggled and still conquered your food demons, and you've never felt better, I promise you'll bring tears to my eyes. That's why I wrote this book.

Please go to my website:

RTIfoods.com/freeyourself

Tell me that you're reaching out because you're reading this book. If you want to have a personal dialog, I'll happily engage.

I wrote this book because I want more people to have what they never thought they could, and that's a healthy relationship with food. I want you to have your life back!

Finally, to all the people for whom this book has touched their soul, or told their story, remember, life is a journey in which we're often lucky enough to participate in creating the road map. I want to leave you with this favorite line from a Tim McGraw song, Better Than I Used to Be:

"I ain't as good as I'm gonna get, but I'm better than I used to be."

Made in the USA
Monee, IL
27 August 2022

12682516R00090